The AIDS Cult

Essays on the Gay Health Crisis

John Lauritsen & Ian Young
Editors

ASKLEPIOS
Provincetown
1997

The AIDS Cult: *Essays on the gay health crisis*

Edited by John Lauritsen & Ian Young

Published by ASKLEPIOS, an imprint of Pagan Press.

"Pagan" is used here to signify the outlook of classical antiquity.

Cover: Rembrandt's etching and drypoint, *Abraham's sacrifice* (1655), is in the Rembrandt House in Amsterdam.

Correspondence regarding this book should be sent to the publisher:

John Lauritsen, Publisher
ASKLEPIOS
Box 1902
Provincetown
MA 02657-0245

If not available in a convenient bookstore, *The AIDS Cult* can be ordered from the publisher at the above address. The price of $15 includes surface postage in the U.S. For overseas airmail add another $8.00. (Payment must be in U.S. dollars — either a check drawn on a U.S. bank or an international money order.)

Library of Congress Catalog Card No. 96-79334
ISBN 0-943742-10-2

CONTENTS

Illustrations:

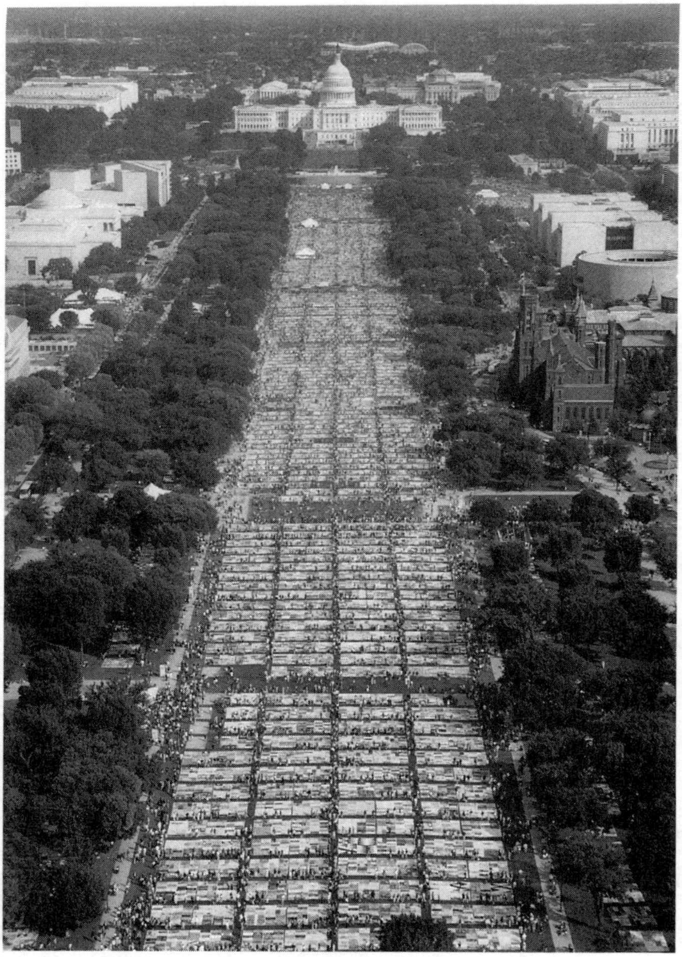

The AIDS Quilt as viewed from the Washington Monument, 11-13 October 1996. The photograph was taken by Paul Margolies and supplied by the Names Project Foundation, according to whose information the Quilt is:

> the largest on-going community arts project in the world. Each of the 32,000 colorful panels in the Quilt was made to remember the life a person lost to AIDS. Panels are 3 feet by 6 feet — the size of a human grave.... Each horizontal row contains 256 individual panels.

Introduction

As this book goes to press, one of its editors is preparing to go to Washington, D.C. for what may be the last display (in its entirety) of the massive Names Project "quilt". The Quilt's panels (how many thousands are there now?) commemorate some of those — mostly gay men — who have died of "AIDS", a disease which, in America at least, is always written in capitals.

Spreading the whole quilt is becoming more and more difficult, simply because the Republic is running out of public spaces vast enough for all the lovingly-crafted memorial panels to be displayed together (like the Nazca Lines, they can only be seen in their entirety from a helicopter). Casper Schmidt, who was one of the first to investigate "the group-fantasy origins of AIDS", compared the Quilt to a *tzompantli,* the Aztec hill of skulls laid out for the gods to witness. Perhaps the New Mexico desert will be the next quilt stop; Bill Clinton did promise a "Manhattan Project for AIDS."

The eight contributors to this collection have varied backgrounds and different vantage points. All of them agree that the orthodox view of our protracted health crisis — as a highly infectious contagion from without — has been found wanting, and that we must seek the causes of this and other medical dilemmas in our own society, our own assumptions, our group-fantasies, our regimens, our recreations, and our rituals.

What really causes AIDS? A virus from Africa? Or our own neglect — or worse — of whole categories of our population? We live in a materialist age, and materialist science has become our religion. But communism is only the first of its churches to collapse. Another — colossal, seemingly impregnable, defensive, tottering — is the gigantic, ramshackle (and expensive) edifice that is orthodox, allopathic medicine. Influenced by the Orient, we are beginning a return to a more holistic approach, one that considers mind as well as microbes. But the sacrifice has not yet ended; the number of panels in the quilt continues to grow.

The AIDS Cult shows how a number of different beliefs, group interests and social forces conspire to make us "sick". This is not a conspiracy in the sense of a conscious plot, but in the original, more profound, sense of a "breathing with" — breathing the same mental atmosphere, sharing the same assumptions, mutually benefitting, and so, collaborating, toward an unconsciously desired result. If we are to analyze our situation properly, we cannot afford to ignore these crucial factors. If we are to solve the case, we must investigate *all* the evidence.

The essays in *The AIDS Cult* offer a fresh, radical view of what the poet E.A. Lacey called "this spell" — the health crisis of our society, as manifested in the gay community. The contributors propose that we reexamine our assumptions about AIDS and terminate the mass sacrificial ritual we have been enacting.

It's time to break away from the dogmas and fantasies that have impeded our understanding, and to recognize what we are doing.

Stop the sacrifice.

Burn the Quilt!

Ian Young
Toronto
October 1996

Preface

A growing number of scientists and others have rejected the HIV-Causes-AIDS hypothesis, as well as the basic concept of "AIDS": that it is a new and coherent disease entity, caused by an infectious microbe and characterized by a narrowly defined state of immune deficiency.

The surveillance definition of "AIDS", constructed by the Centers for Disease Control (CDC), contains so many internal contradictions and has been revised so many times, that one may justifiably deny the very existence of "AIDS". What do undeniably exist, however, are the many illnesses associated with the syndrome, and it is part of our task, as critics of the orthodox AIDS paradigm, to explain the occurrence of these illnesses in a small subset of gay men.

Up to now we AIDS critics have tended to slight the psychosocial factors that are damaging the health of gay men — and the HIV believers have ignored them completely. The essays in this book should redress the balance. They examine the irrational, *cultic* aspects of the AIDS phenomenon.

About the contributors to *The AIDS Cult:*

My co-editor, Ian Young, is a poet living in Toronto. He has been active in the gay liberation movement since the 60s, as an activist, writer and publisher. Among his many books are *The AIDS Dissidents: An annotated bibliography* (1993) and *The Stonewall Experiment* (1995).

I, John Lauritsen, a retired survey research analyst, now live in Provincetown after 32 years in New York City. I've been in gay liberation since the 60s and am the proprietor of Pagan Press (founded 1982). My books include *Poison By Prescription: The AZT Story* (1990) and *The AIDS War* (1993).

The late Casper Schmidt, MD was born and raised in what is now called Namibia. He had a psychoanalytic practice in New York City, and was Associate Director of the Institute of Psychohistory.

George Hazlehurst, MD is an internist living in Arizona. Since 1973 he has carried on research in psychosomatic medicine, exploring the unconscious mind to inquire into primal cause/cure of disease states. He is convinced that cure of cancers and other puzzling diseases, including AIDS, can never be found so long as patients' beliefs, attitudes, and emotions are ignored by science.

Michael Ellner, living in New York City, is President of the alternative AIDS organization, Health Education AIDS Liaison (HEAL). He is a master hypnotherapist.

Andrew Cort, also a leading member of HEAL, is a practising chiropractor and nutritionist, who now resides in Barrington, Rhode Island.

Cass Mann lives near London, where for many years he has been the guiding light of Positively Healthy — an organization which has enabled hundreds of people with diagnoses of "AIDS" or "HIV-positive" to regain their health and remain healthy. He was an organizer of the international conference, "AZT On Trial" (London, June 1993).

The late Michael Callen was a singer and song writer, and a founder and leader of the People With AIDS Coalition. His book, *Surviving AIDS,* was published in 1990.

Much of the inspiration for this book comes from Casper Schmidt, whose counsel was of great benefit to me during the years I knew him. On a number of occasions we discussed how to bring his ideas to a wider audience. Having observed with dismay the systematic and all-pervasive censorship of viewpoints that challenged the AIDS Establishment, we agreed that finding a major publisher was unlikely, and he assured me I was more than welcome to publish anything he had written on AIDS. I am happy that I can at last fulfill my promise to him by republishing his seminal essay, "The Group-Fantasy Origins of AIDS".

If he were still alive, Casper would have volunteered to design the cover. He was a fine artist, whose African-motif paintings had whimsy and flair. In particular I remember his ironical rendition of "St. Sebastian", which could have been the basis of the cover. Unfortunately, the painting's whereabouts is unknown.

As it is, I think Casper would have liked the Rembrandt etching and the Old Dutch typeface used for the cover. (He had a keen interest in typography.) And he would have been very pleased with the other essays in *The AIDS Cult.*

The message of the Rembrandt — and the sentiment shared by all of the contributors to this book — is that the sacrifice must cease. We are doing what we can to end it, but our forces are limited, and we need all the help we can get.

John Lauritsen
Provincetown
October 1996

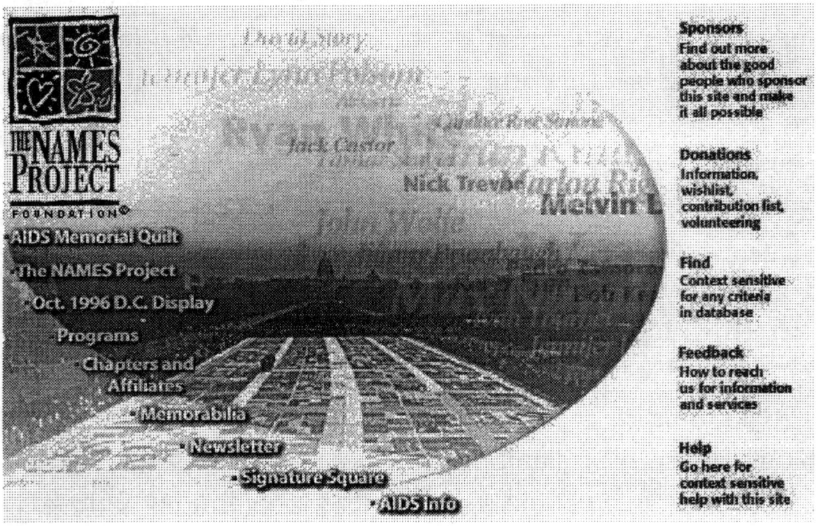

The home page logo of the Names Project web site on the Internet (http://www.aidsquilt.org/). A "major sponsor", among the "good people who sponsor this site", is Stadtlanders Pharmacy ("the nation's leading specialty pharmacy, meeting the needs of individuals living with challenging health conditions....") No doubt Stadtlanders dispensed prescriptions for AZT and similar drugs to a great many of those commemorated by the Quilt.

According to the Names Project web site:

> Without walkways, the Quilt spans the equivalent of 14 football fields and weighs 44 tons. With walkways, the Quilt spans 22 football fields and weighs 50 tons. Over 50 new panels are added every week.

CHAPTER I

The Group-Fantasy Origins of AIDS[1]

Casper G. Schmidt

Since 1981 a noteworthy epidemic of an acquired immune deficiency syndrome (AIDS) has been described in the larger part of the First World, beginning with the United States of America, but now also found in Western Europe, South and Central Africa, Australia and a scattering of other pockets. It has been described mostly in a few select groups of people at greater risk: homosexual men, IV drug abusers, Haitians and Africans, children of people in at-risk groups, and a small percentage of people who fit into none of these categories. At the time of the writing of this paper (July, 1984), the total number of U.S. cases reported to the Centers for Disease Control in Atlanta is in excess of 5,200, of whom approximately 45 per cent have died.

Though small in scope, this epidemic is intensely cathected, as are all group-fantasy rituals. (This is in contrast with Alzheimer's disease, for example, which is unconnected to group-fantasy and kills 120,000 people per year.)

The most popular scientific theory about the etiology of AIDS is a viral hypothesis. According to this theory — which has been taken over by the lay press — AIDS is caused by a novel or mutated virus spread through the exchange of body fluids or through infected needles. A suitable candidate for this viral agent

---

[1]Originally published in *The Journal of Psychohistory,* Summer 1984.

was discovered by French researchers who published their findings in May of 1983. There was very little media attention paid to this since the information was at that time out of sync with the dominant group-fantasy in the U.S. By the spring of 1984 American researchers announced identification of a similar retrovirus (HTLV-III), with a formal press conference and a great deal of media attention. Immediately after this the consensus of mainstream America was that AIDS had been "solved", with a blood test soon to be available (however uncertain its significance and shaky its interpretation), and with optimistic predictions of a vaccine soon to emerge from the laboratory.

There are, however, not one but *two* main classes of contagious illness in man: infectious diseases (spread by germs) and contagious forms of psychological disturbances (spread by suggestion). It is often forgotten that the reigning theories of the origins of infectious illness before Pasteur came along were those of humoral causation ("bad humors") and the theory of putrefaction. It took Pasteur years to prove and convince people of the germ theory of infection. Once that explanation became accepted, it became unshakable due to the inertia of the mind. To this day, every single disease entity for which no adequate explanation has been found has been ascribed to a viral origin (from schizophrenia down through autoimmune disorders).

I propose an alternative hypothesis for the etiology of AIDS, based on the second of these two mechanisms of contagion in man. This will posit a psychosocial origin of epidemic AIDS, which will lie on the cusp between immunology, pathology and psychology (the latter including the psychology of both individuals and groups). I will do so in twin papers meant to be read in tandem: this one, which will deal mostly with the group psychology, and a second paper for the medical press. In the medical paper, which is entitled, "The Pathogenesis of Epidemic AIDS", I account for the "biological" end of the disorder. It will trace the physiological effects of the group-psychological factors outlined in this paper on the individual patient, with the resultant epidemic of severe, mostly masked, reactive depression in the at-risk groups, of which the immune deficiency is one facet. It will outline the pathway and the mechanism by which the cell-mediated immunity may be suppressed, and will provide an animal model for AIDS, as I discuss below.

HYPOTHESIS

In this paper I would like to present the evidence available to me in support of the hypothesis:

(a) that AIDS is a typical example of *epidemic hysteria*;

(b) that the epidemic has at its core an unconscious group delusion, which can be called the *group-fantasy of scapegoating*, according to which the poison feelings of the entire group are injected into containers who are called scapegoats and whose destruction rids the group of these bad feelings and insures its purification of guilt and sinfulness;

(c) that the same *fantasy complex* underlies this scapegoating ritual as was found for leprosy during the Middle Ages and early Renaissance;

(d) that the proximal and distal causes of the tensions giving rise to the epidemic can be found in the *group psychology* of the United States and (to a lesser extent, inasmuch as they follow the cultural lead of America) the West since World War II;

(e) that among the more important *distal causes* are the effects of the following drastic changes in cultural ethos: the development of nuclear arsenals with a potential for obliterating the world, and the changes this has forced in the psychology of warfare; the introduction of birth control and the invention of "recreational sex"; positive changes in the mental health of American women over the last 35 to 40 years, culminating in the women's liberation movement and the proposed Equal Rights Amendment to the U.S. Constitution; and the "liberation" of various disenfranchised groups such as blacks and homosexuals;

(f) that the *proximal cause* can be found in a vast, society-wide conservative swing (or neo-populist trend) in public opinion since 1977, culminating in the Reagan years and the Central American conflict;

(g) that the combination of these unconscious group tensions brought about a subtle and sophisticated, but nevertheless *sacrificial witch hunt*, in which the participants were the Moral Majority and an assortment of other conservative groups (as hunters) and the nation's drug addicts and homosexuals (as hunted);

(h) that both of these subgroups are *acting-out* group-sanctioned and *group-delegated* rôles, which acting-out takes place mostly outside of awareness;

(i) that these attacks resulted in an *epidemic of depression* based mostly on shame;

(j) that the core sign of AIDS, the *reduction of cell-mediated immunity*, is one of the typical vegetative signs of a severe depression (the mechanism of which will be the focus of the medical companion piece to this paper);

(k) that the epidemic represents, in the group's unconscious fantasies, an *equivalent of war*, during which the group keeps careful count of the sacrifices;

(l) that most of the members of the group (the U.S.A.) are in a regression vis-à-vis this phenomenon, a *trance state* which is noticeable in a certain suspension of logic in the lay press and in the medical literature;

(m) that there are powerful forces at work to delay the solution of the puzzle posed by this epidemic and to obscure its group-fantasy origins, since the *epidemic itself is a wished-for solution* to pre-existing conflicts;

(n) and finally that, since the epidemic is psychogenic, the prediction can be made that the group will decide when it should be over (when they have "had enough"), a decision which will be broadcast to the group members through the media, so that after a suitable lag period (based on the time needed for the T-helper lymphocytes to be restored to previous levels of functioning) the epidemic will resolve and the *incidence will descend from epidemic to endemic* levels.

EPIDEMIC HYSTERIA

The capacity for effective working-through of emotional conflicts within groups is restricted. Bion has shown how groups have great difficulty in performing real work, and how insidious and predominant are those emotional positions which he called basic assumptions (where fantasy solutions hold sway over realistic ones). The commonest pathway for the discharge of dammed-up group tension, historically speaking, is recourse to action. Thus the regular occurrence of human sacrifice, ritual scapegoating, cannibalism, and war throughout history, even though these rituals become more covert the closer one gets to the present. The group actions need not necessarily be destructive, and reparative rituals such as baby booms are also found (usually as a guilt-motivated attempt at replacing those "babies" that had been ritually killed off in fantasy during war).

Opposed to these instances of group action, where the direction of discharge lies outward, there is a second avenue of discharge in which the aggression is turned inward. This gives rise to waves of psychological and psychosomatic disturbances, to which the descriptive label of ***epidemic hysteria*** has been given. These occur in group members of lower status or in those who do not wield much power (predominantly women, children, laborers, prisoners, and other "powerless" members of the group).

Some solid reviews of the reported cases and the literature have appeared. Since 1943 there has been an upsurge in interest in this topic, after a long hiatus since 1917 during which it virtually disappeared from all medical writing.[1] However, in the mainstream of American psychiatry very little attention has been paid to these phenomena. For example, in the *Comprehensive Textbook of Psychiatry* by Freedman, Kaplan and Sadock (Second Edition, 1975) — surely the most catholic and eclectic textbook ever devised — I find but one reference to the concept of mass hysteria. Slater and Roth's *Clinical Psychiatry* (1972) has two, both pertaining to children. (My interpretation is that there may be a strong unconscious resistance to the examination of one's own group participation: since it is both frightening and awesome, and, when known, such awareness interferes with one's ability to act out the group rituals.)

To turn now to the phenomenology of epidemic hysteria. The duration of the episodes so far recorded are all relatively short (ranging from a few hours to a few months, only Markush[2] boldly including lengthier ones). The prototypical epidemic is as follows: in a social situation of pronounced stressfulness, in which the members have little or no recourse (schools, factories), a particular stressor is added to the mix; after this a few persons develop vague, non-specific somatic complaints, which go undetected; soon more people become ill; it comes to the attention of the authorities (management and medical), and a rumor spreads, ascribing the outbreak to some toxin in the environment; the group becomes polarized into those who help versus those who fall ill; all stops are pulled out (a typical scene has a panic-stricken school surrounded by fire engines and ambulances with sirens whining, medical epidemiologists taking air and water samples, while school girls are fainting all over) and everything is enveloped in an atmosphere of crisis; the local media spread the news and the rumor, thus precipitating further attacks; an intervention is made (such as closing the school); gradually the number of casualties declines, and the epidemic disappears as mysteriously as it had come.

This can be schematically illustrated (with all the morphological features named in bold print) by a recent outbreak which was extensively and elegantly investigated by Kerckhoff and Back.[3]

The June Bug Epidemic

In Spartanburg, South Carolina, an epidemic occurred in June, 1962 at a large textile plant. There were many sources of strain within the plant: lots of overtime had been put in; many of the workers earned half or more of the income of their respective families; there were strained relationships with supervisors and concerns over work output; in addition, many workers showed role-conflict denial, or a lack of concern that their overtime work kept them from their families *(distal causes)*. June was a particularly busy month, when production was at a peak for the fall line *(proximal cause)*. For about three weeks people had been complaining of bugs and of being bitten, and one week before the epidemic started the plant had been sprayed three times with malathion (the *"silent" penumbra* of the epidemic). On Friday one person became ill, complaining of severe nausea, and had to be treated by the company physician. Five more got ill on the Tuesday following, fainting and breaking out in hives all over so that some even had to be hospitalized (*core syndrome* of the epidemic). There was a widespread belief that people were getting ill after being bitten by a poisonous bug, introduced into the plant on cotton from England on that Wednesday *(belief in a poison threat)*. The spread of cases was as shown (Figure 1). On Wednesday the plant was closed down and fumigated. (This was the unconscious *epidemic aim*, which resolved all tensions related to the work situation through simple avoidance.) Over the next few days the plant opened again, with workers returning in an agitated state. Various experts and authorities were called in (health officials, entomologists, representatives from the plant's insurance and the local exterminating company) and samples of food, bugs and air were taken. More cases occurred on Friday, on Saturday and the next Monday, after which the episode ceased. The time from the onset of the penumbra to the onset of the core syndrome (*penumbral lead time*) was three weeks, and the duration of the core syndrome itself was 11 days. Two months later, when the researchers investigated the epidemic, 51% of the unaffected expressed a belief in "the bug" as the cause of the disturbance, while 81% of those affected thought so (*extent of the belief* in the poison threat). In their analysis of the dynamics of the epidemic, the investigators found that 75% of those affected could be predicted by a few variables: (a) strain (the more strain, the more likely persons were to be affected); (b) social influence (if workers knew two or more affected cases, they were more likely to fall ill themselves); and (c) denial (which increased the likelihood of becoming affected in all categories). They found that the *psychic contagion* (the belief that people were getting ill from the bite of the bug) spread by imitation, by suggestion and by personal contact:

> In any such case there are several processes of dissemination going on at the same time, all of which are interrelated but any one or combination of which may become the focus of attention: (1) the spread of a belief in a threat; (2) the spread of the experience of symptoms; (3) the spread of relatively unobtrusive methods of coping with the threat and/or the symptoms; (4) the spread of cases of collapse in the face of the threat and/or the experience of symptoms via seeking medical aid.

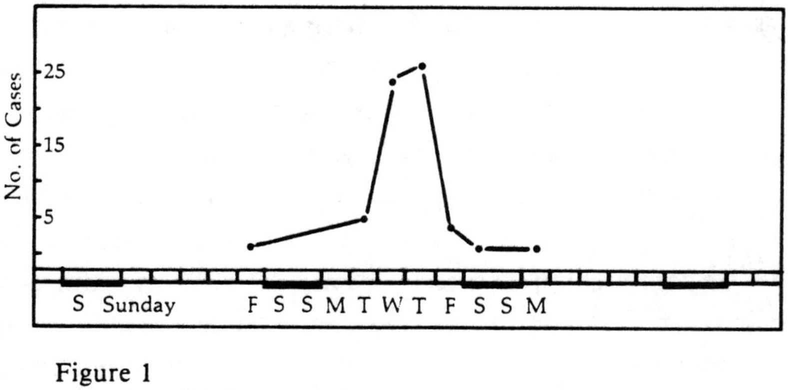

Figure 1
June Bug epidemic: incidence of cases

The most promising approach to the complex phenomenon of epidemic hysteria is from a psychoanalytic point of view, of which Sirois is the foremost and most eloquent proponent.[4] (Trying to understand group dynamics of this kind without the conceptual tools such as "the unconscious" and "group-fantasy" is self-limiting, like trying to understand diabetes without recourse to concepts such as "molecule" and "blood sugar".) Central to his theory and also that of most social psychologists working with such epidemics, is the idea of an unconscious belief shared by many (a group-fantasy). Sirois theorizes that these epidemics represent a contagious type of psychopathology, where the contagion is "a wish whose vector is a fantasy that circulates in a reservoir of susceptible persons".[5] He defines three elements of the epidemic: a prodrome, an epidemic moment (when first cases become manifest), and a rebound (or secondary waves of affliction). For each episode, he says, there is an underlying fantasy which is cathartically worked-through via the epidemic disturbance. An epidemic of hysteria develops (as opposed to other forms of disturbance) due to three factors: (a) the group regression; (b) identification with the index cases; and (c) the unconscious nature of the underlying conflicts or fantasies. "This last aspect is a crucial factor in fostering the manifestation of the conflict through displaced, symbolic or alternate channels."[6] Thus, he argues, the psychosomatic presentation of most epidemics.

The biggest theoretical challenge to the researchers, and the aspect most resistant to explanation or to plausible hypotheses, is the simple fact that perfectly normal and seemingly healthy people get caught up in these epidemics. The disconcerting possibility that this raises is that we are all susceptible. When the psychometricians measure the subjects they find nothing to explain why certain people with a certain make-up get sick and others with identical profiles do not. The tools used to measure them are, however, those designed for picking up individual psychopathology, often of a gross kind. It seems to me that they are measuring the wrong thing. To state it by analogy: if one were to try to determine, in a crowded disco, which people would get up to dance to a certain number, the highest probabilities found would lie on an intersect between the person's drive state (how strong the urge is to dance) and some particular characteristic (what a specific song or partner means to a specific person). Thus, what is sought to be measured here is something inherently evanescent. In an epidemic of hysteria these variables would seem to be (a) the strength of the propensity to get sick in a psychosomatic way (a conversion factor), and (b) the specific contents of the group-fantasies and how well they fit the fantasy structure of the individual (so that the same person would be susceptible to a dancing mania but not susceptible to an epidemic of depression).

In time all of these epidemics come to be organized around — and retrospectively explained by — a core fantasy, which may be called the ***fantasy of a poison threat***. It belongs to the psychology of belief systems, and we have to look to the dynamics of delusions for an explanation. Just as with individuals, the delusions shared by groups are reparative mechanisms: attempts at making sense out of inchoate or incoherent preverbal or affective experiences, or out of a painful and poorly understood reality. As such they come after the fact, once the disturbance is already well under way. In most instances where the formation of delusions has been studied extensively (see Frosch[7] and Arieti[8], the person experiences a sudden and remarkable sense of relief once the delusion is formed. The confusion subsides.[9] Especially in hypochondriacal and melancholic delusions, the formation of the delusion and its psychosomatic expression permits massive relief from psychotic anxieties. Sperling[10] found that psychosomatic symptoms are solutions for anxieties of psychotic intensity. When conversion symptoms are "released" from their somatic form, they reveal intense and terrifying, and usually psychotic symptoms.[11] And in an epidemic of hysteria the delusion of a poison threat becomes the organizer for tremendous amounts of "poison feelings".

This shared fantasy of a poison threat is found in all cases of epidemic hysteria where there is enough information, and my hypothesis is that it will prove true for all cases if properly studied. These fantasies are culture-specific in contents (based on the theory of disease for each culture), and syntonic with the rest of the cultural beliefs. Underlying these various contents there is a universal radical which remains cross-culturally the same: in all epidemics the bad feelings are ascribed to some contact with poison or a poison threat.

During the twentieth century, since most epidemics take place in schools or factories, and in keeping with the dominant theories of disease, these epidemics are thought to be caused by: Poison gas, mystery gas, anesthetic gas, strange odors, acid or acrid smells, contaminated air, radioactive fall-out, poisonous dyes, fumes and solvents, and to on, in monotonous profusion. And despite extensive toxicological work-ups, no evidence for any of these toxins is ever found. (Suffice it to say that I exclude all cases of genuine poisoning.)

In other times, other fantasy poisons are found. In medieval Spain through Nazi Germany, Jews were believed to poison wells, or were blood poisoners of the group, or the Devil sent his assistants to poison the wells.[12] In southern Italy people were "bitten" by poisonous tarantulas, thus poisoning their blood for life, a fate which could only be countered by dancing each summer until they dropped from exhaustion, after which they were bled (removal of "poison blood").[13] The dancers in the dancing manias of the Middle Ages believed they were dancing in rivers of blood, so that they had to lift their feet high.[14] In East Africa people caught up in a running mania were trying to escape from imaginary radio-active fall-out.[15] During the Salem witch trials the witches were beaten with imaginary whips until the floor of the court was covered with imaginary ("poison") blood.[16] In epidemics of "Dhat syndrome" in India and South East Asia, men's semen became spoiled through their being libertines, and this spoiled semen (fantasy of poison sperm) had to be countered by celibacy and other restrictions on sexual activity.[17] In an epidemic of koro in Thailand, it was thought that the retraction of the genitals was caused by Thai food (noodles and cigarettes) being poisoned by Vietnamese refugees.[18]

A most significant finding is that these epidemics follow the divisions of class, ethnic groups and other cultural differences. (This is one of the major distinguishing features between epidemics of infection and epidemics of hysteria, since the former does not display this "ability" to follow cultural "fault lines".) Thus, in an epidemic in a Singapore factory, Malay workers were predominantly affected, while those of different ethnic groups who became affected, were few and showed only mild, transient symptoms.[19] In the June Bug epidemic outlined above, the poisonous insect bit only white women working on the morning shift, while other workers on other shifts went unaffected through the same "contaminated" space. Among the Australian aborigines depression tends to occur in clusters rather than in individuals, and when this happens it will, for example, affect all the classificatory brothers of a clan in unison.[20] The line between those affected and those left untouched can therefore be said to follow the cleavage lines of self, self-perception and identity.

Another frequently encountered finding is the fantasy that the poison which caused the epidemic was introduced from outside. It is obvious from analyses of these epidemics that tensions and unresolved conflicts originate from within the group. When these factors, which are psychologically speaking "poisoning the workplace", cannot consciously be identified and reasonably dealt with (due to denial or other defense mechanisms), they are projected outwards. Thus the poison threat is nearly always seen as coming from at least outside of the individual. When more severe regressions occur, the threat is seen as coming from farther away: in the June bug epidemic the culprits were thought to be poisonous insects that had arrived on cloth from England.

Once the epidemic has progressed to the point of consolidation — i.e., once the group delusion about its cause has been formed and disseminated — it thereafter dictates which measures will have to be taken to combat it. This can be called the *epidemic aim*. Like all things form the unconscious, these measures, though they may seem believable and imperative, are naive and concrete. The most popular solution is to locate the poison — in fantasy — and then to avoid it by closing down the school or factory, or to build a *cordon sanitaire* around it (protective isolation), or to expel it to the outside of the group (e.g. by sending people into exile, such as Castro's Mariel evacuation). The core fantasy is always one of poison being contained through the epidemic aim in a person or a place (which may also be a fetish object), and then to avoid direct contact with it, since the poison is thought to spread by touch.

Not all people who come to participate in the epidemic share the epidemic disturbance to the same extent. This is most clearly seen in the 1944 epidemic of the "phantom anesthetist" of Mattoon, Illinois.[21] As shown in Figure 2, two principal beliefs were registered: the one belief was that there was a prowler going around people's back yards; the second was the fantasy of people being put to sleep by a phantom anesthetist squirting gas through people's bedroom windows. This difference is found in most of the epidemics for which enough information is available.

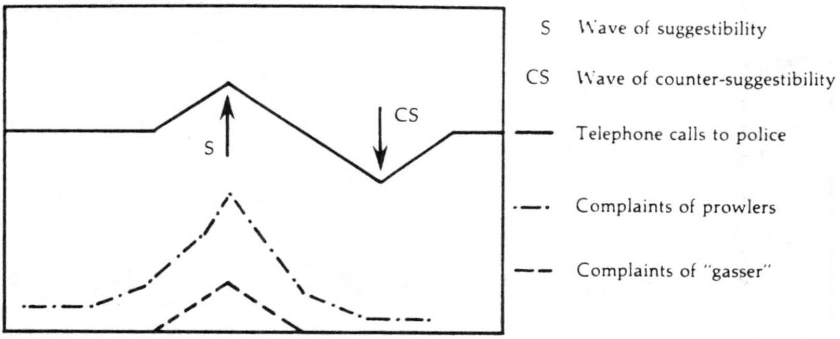

Figure 2
The "Phantom Anesthetist" of Mattoon, Illinois

I propose that these fantasies be separated in principle into a core and a "silent" penumbra (as I indicated above in the synopsis of the June Bug epidemic). The penumbral syndrome is found in those who share in the group disturbance — and thus the group delusion — to a more limited degree than those with the core syndrome. I ascribe this difference to varying degrees of resistance to suggestion that people show within the group situation. In AIDS, this separation into a core and a penumbral syndrome is clear, as can be seen from the graph depicting the incidence of AIDS and of amebiasis (a syndrome of diarrhea caused by an intestinal parasite) in San Francisco. It is my thesis that amebiasis (as also later the lymphadenopathy syndrome, or general swelling of the lymph glands) constitutes the penumbral syndrome (figure 3). I take the differential factor to be a quantitative one, with amebiasis resulting from a lesser reduction of the cell-mediated immunity than that required to develop the full AIDS syndrome.

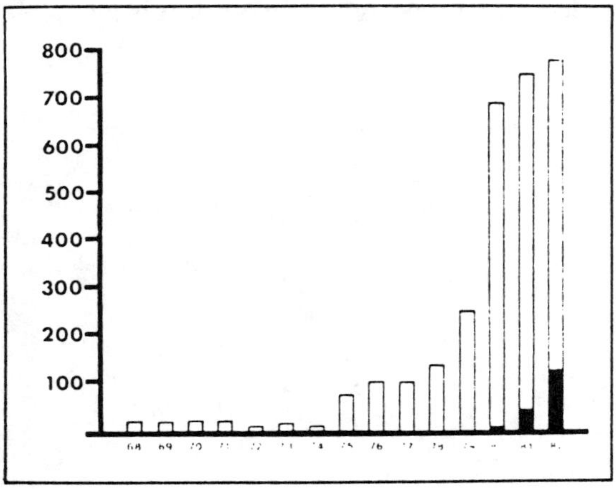

Figure 3
Annual Incidence: AIDS & Amebiasis (San Francisco)[22]

□ AMEBIASIS
■ AIDS

A final point concerning phenomenology. As Johnson was the first to identify, and as can be seen in Figure 2, the typical case of epidemic hysteria occurs in the form of two waves: a wave of suggestibility which is replaced by a wave of countersuggestibility, after which the whole system returns to a baseline condition. During that epidemic back yard noises, which otherwise would have seemed incidental, were ascribed — under the impact of this wave of suggestibility — to prowlers and later to the phantom anesthetist. After this wave had passed, identical noises were passed over as insignificant. The actual epidemic is parallel to the wave of suggestibility, and the wave of countersuggestibility gives rise to an unusually quiet and peaceful period afterwards. Within the wave of suggestibility there is a symmetry, so that the first part of the epidemic to appear (the penumbra) is the last to disappear, which symmetry also holds true for the core syndrome.

We can therefore come to a definition. Epidemic hysteria is (a) a form of collective mental disorder that takes place in a susceptible population, (b) through the mechanism of a contagion which spreads by suggestion; (c) this susceptibility is defined by the interface between individual character structure (drives) and distal group tensions, (d) and is enhanced by proximal stressors; (e) the contagion can be a wish, a fantasy or a delusion or whatever kind, (f) and gives rise through somatization to somatic or psychosomatic symptoms, (g) the purpose of which is to resolve conflicts through primary process (or unconscious) means, since (h) direct, conscious expression and resolution of conflict is impossible due to group defenses; (i) the spread increases geometrically since the occurrence of the first cases confirms the unconscious fantasy of a poison threat, (j) which is the unconscious encoding of bad feelings projected outwards, (k) in a fantasy complex syntonic with the culture, (l) which comes to be shared by various members of the group to various degrees, giving rise to a core and penumbral syndromes; (m) it is self-limiting, since the epidemic disturbance permits discharge of pent-up tensions (n) and the mobilization of the rest of the group in a reparative role.

It is my interpretation that the gestalt of AIDS, in its epidemic form, fits this definition precisely. According to this interpretation, the viral etiology which is subscribed to by many should be seen as part of the unconscious group delusion of a poison threat. The evidence presented so far supports the view that the virus which has been discovered (LAV/HTLV-III) is probably just another opportunistic infection, and plays, if at all, only a late role in the causal chain of AIDS. As in other epidemics, the poison which "causes" the disorder is assumed to originate from outside the country. At first it was thought that the poison had been brought back to the U.S. by vacationing homosexuals from Haiti.[23] The final parts of the fantasy — that the virus was spread in Africa by "itinerant inoculators" and had traveled from there to the U.S. via Haiti — was definitively formulated by Jacques Leibowitch of France, in a book entitled *Un virus étrange venue d'ailleurs (A Strange Virus From Elsewhere,* published in April 1984).[24] The route of the poison is clearly shown on this map from *Newsweek* (Figure 4).[25]

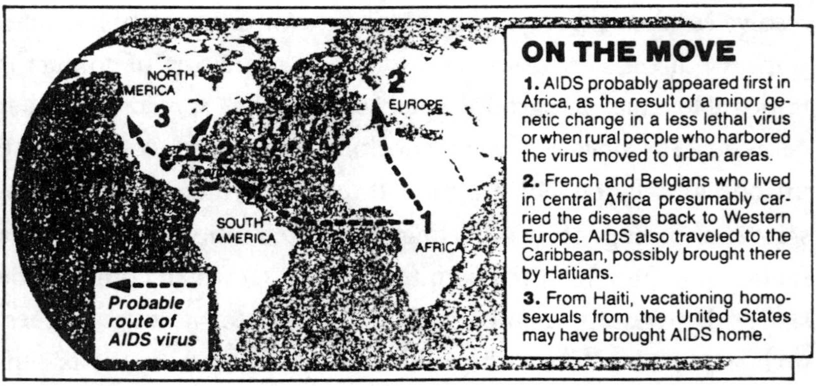

Figure 4
"Proof" that the poison comes from elsewhere

The unconscious social conflict which AIDS is called upon to resolve is twofold: (a) unconscious drug-taking and homosexual fantasies within the general population, brought dangerously close to the surface because of the permissiveness of the 60s and 70s. The bad feelings stirred up by these changes were projected outwards, and into the scapegoats; and (b) guilt over sexual and addictive excesses within the general population as well as within these two subcultures. As we shall see below, when all of America swung to the right and became more righteous and dogmatic (taking a stand against license and permissiveness), a superego position was delegated to the New Right. They delivered a harangue to shame those who represented parts of ourselves (the id) which we now disavowed. This created a wave of reactive depression, caused by repression of the retaliatory fury that the shamed person feels. Three group-fantasies of a poison threat were evolved along the way, which in turn confirmed the delusional thinking and accelerated the epidemic. In fantasy, AIDS was thought to be caused by (a) promiscuity or, in the case of drug addicts, the abuse of drugs (fantasy of moral corruption and decay); (b) viruses contained in blood and blood products (fantasy of poison blood), and (c) viruses contained in bodily fluids, especially sperm (fantasy of poison sperm). These fantasies dictated the epidemic aims: (a) to reduce sexual activity or drug use to the point of abstinence or celibacy (at least in fantasy); (b) to stop the exchange of bodily fluids through the use of condoms, masturbation clubs, "safe sex" and sex rings of "clean" partners; and (c) to avoid the giving or receiving of blood. The core syndrome is the official definition of AIDS by the Centers for Disease Control in Atlanta, while the penumbral syndromes include the epidemic incidence of amebiasis (part of the "Gay Bowel Syndrome"), the lymphadenopathy syndrome and various *forms frustes* of depression. As I report elsewhere, a joke has come into circulation on every one of these facets of the group psychology.[26] The group trance is at this point heavily upon us, and anyone who proposes that AIDS is not caused by the virus (equivalent, in terms of the June Bug epidemic, to someone saying there was no bug) is viewed as a threat to the group's solidarity.

I have charted in Table I the major features of AIDS and the epidemic of the June Bug, to point up the parallels.

TABLE I
Comparison: AIDS & June Bug Epidemics

	June Bug epidemic	*AIDS epidemic*
Distal Causes:	Strains: overtime, half or more of family income, worry over output, supervisor Role-conflict denial	Gender dysphoria: women's & gay liberation, ERA, birth control & sexual revolutions, curbs on warfare
Proximal Causes:	Peak of production	Conservative swing & clampdown on permissiveness
Time Spread:		
(a) penumbral lead:	?3 weeks	6 years (1975 - 1981)
(b) core halflife	6 days	?5 years (1981 - 1984?)
Scapegoat Fantasies:		
(a) hunters (superego position)	Management	New Right, Moral Majority, conservative Christians
(b) hunted (id position)	White female workers on first shift	Pleasure seekers (drug addicts & homosexuals)
Clinical Presentation:		
(a) core syndrome	Insect bites with severe nausea, vomiting, hives and fainting	Overt depression, lowered cell-mediated immunity with opportunistic infections & Kaposi's sarcoma
(b) silent penumbra	Complaints about insect bites, anxiety	Lymphadenopathy syndrome, amebiasis, masked depression
Group Delusion:		
(a) poison threat	Poisonous bug in cloth	Poison sperm, poison blood & dangerous promiscuity
(b) origin of poison	England	Africa

The group-fantasies in America contained virtually no mention of the other, officially defined at-risk groups, and there was a reluctance to include them in the official list of risk groups (especially in the case of children, since scapegoating fantasies about children provoke intense guilt). My interpretation it that people in these other risk groups have become involved through a spill-over effect on the basis of unusual suggestibility or because of an unconscious identification with one of the risk groups. Children are a special case. In the medical paper I hypothesize that these children suffer from severe anaclitic depression (through deprivation or neglect), and that the pathophysiological mechanism is identical to that in adult patients with AIDS.

The fantasy complex of AIDS (i.e. the triad of promiscuity, poison blood, poison sperm) is not new. It is identical to the one in vogue during the Middle Ages to explain the origins of leprosy. It was generally accepted that leprosy was associated with violent sexual excitement and moral impurity — by the nineteenth century it was common opinion that leprosy was the consequence of lust. During the Middle Ages leprosy was thought to follow from the "filth of lechery", the "impurity of lust"[27] (fantasy of dangerous promiscuity). A second cause for leprosy was "the conception of a child 'in menstrual tyme'" (fantasy of menstrual, i.e. poisonous, blood).[28] A third group of etiological ideas are fantasies of poisonous sperm: John of Gaddesden warns that a man who sleeps with a woman who has previously had intercourse with a leper will contract the disease.[29] Bernard Gordon adds that the man will become leprous only if the woman still retains the seminal fluid of the leper.[30] Copland's translation of Guy of Chauliac advises the diagnostician "to enquyre yf he hath had the company of any lepresse woman. And yf lazar [i.e. a leper] had medled with her afore hym and lately because of the infect mater and the contagious filth that she hadde receyved of hym."[30]

It can be seen that this fantasy complex has not changed, and is encountered intact today, except that in the AIDS epidemic the fantasies have been translated into modern idiom (so that "contagious filth" becomes "semen containing cytomegalovirus or HTLV-III" or, more sophisticated still, "immunosuppressive sperm"). These unconscious fantasies are found not only in the lay press, but they determine the direction of our scientific thinking, so that in scientific magazines usually sceptical clinicians subscribe to them without sufficient proof.

THE MYSTERIOUS LEAP FROM THE MIND TO THE BODY

Against the grain of monoetiological thinking and an unconsciously held Cartesian dualism,[32] I posit that AIDS is a bio-psycho-social disorder. I argue that a sequence of group psychological events in the U.S. has shamed — and mercilessly so — the homosexuals and the drug addicts, giving rise to an epidemic of shame-induced depression. (I examine the dynamics of shame in the next section, and the ways by which it was achieved in later sections.)

Now, depression is not simply a psychological disorder. In fact, it is very much the "iceberg of psychiatric disorders", with just as much if not more going on below the level of consciousness than above. In transcultural psychiatry it has been found that the "psychological form of depression" (sadness, guiltiness and weeping) is not often found outside of the First World.[33] (My thesis, based on deMause's history of childrearing modes,[34] is that the psychological style of the upbringing of the child will determine the clinical picture when they become depressed as adults: the more sophisticated the childrearing becomes, the more the typology of depression will be "psychological".) The most common form of depression encountered elsewhere is that of a ***masked depression***, in which the most obvious signs are the absence of pleasure and the various psychosomatic/somatic components of depression (weight loss, anorexia, lassitude, slowing down of movement, amenorrhea: the so-called "vegetative signs" of depression). In the medical paper I present evidence for the hypothesis that AIDS is a form of masked depression, and that a reduction in the cell-mediated immunity is one of the characteristic vegetative signs of a severe depression.

An animal model for AIDS has eagerly been sought, so far without much success, among infected primates (the so-called Simian AIDS). I think that the answer lies in a different direction and that the guidelines used in looking for an animal model have — incorrectly — been based on the infectious disease model. The closest animal equivalent to depression is that of "learned helplessness."[35] When rats are exposed to conditions of inescapable shock in the laboratory, they develop learned helplessness, in which they cease to do anything that would alleviate their suffering. They then go on to develop a syndrome of weight loss, stunted growth, anorexia and a lowering of their cell-mediated immunity.[36] These are the same signs and symptoms found in AIDS (allowing for differences between species), and my hypothesis is that this is the valid animal model for AIDS in humans.

THE GROUP PSYCHOLOGY OF SHAME

Shame is one of the two superego affects (the other being guilt) and is the more problematic of the two. Lewis distinguishes between them as follows:[37] shame is the bad feeling you get when you perceive a defect in what you are, whereas guilt arises from the perception that you have done something wrong. Shame is accompanied by strong autonomic arousal, while guilt, being more "cognitive", has a less intense affective tone.

When the defenses against the experience of shame fail, various emergency measures are called into action, of which there are three germane to our purpose: the first is a wish to remove oneself from the painfulness of the observation which brings about the shame (the "Evil Eye" of folklore), and may include wishes to hide, to bury oneself, to withdraw, or ultimately to remove oneself from the group by way of exile or suicide. The second is a strong retaliatory fury which may be directed at the shamer ("to shame the shamer") or at the self. The more sophisticated the group or the individual, the more these vengeful, retaliatory aggressions are aim-inhibited and turned against the self (causing self-destructive actions, from minor accidents to a fury ending in a flamboyant suicide). Where these self-destructive actings-out are inhibited, the rage gets turned against the self and becomes depression. The third is a libidinization of the retaliatory fury with inappropriate sexual excitement. When this is acted upon, the sexual partner becomes in fantasy the object of the destructive rage. This mechanism is one of the root causes of compulsive sexuality, setting up a pathway which is called into service each time the subject feels ashamed.[38]

The reason for the strong reactions provoked by shame is most cogently explained by Piers:[39] "Behind the feeling of shame stands not the fear of hatred, but the fear of contempt which, on an even deeper level of the unconscious, spells fear of abandonment, the death by emotional starvation." On a social level, within the group dynamics, this becomes the fear of exclusion from the life-blood of the group, and of ostracism, which is the social death of the organism.

The way in which shame is used in a primitive setting is instructive. It is usually done through the delivery of a ***harangue*** (which I propose as the technical term for all shaming procedures). In a small village in Papua-New Guinea, for example, this will be enacted by one person shouting out the harangue at night, and it is listened to by all in absolute silence. The accused individual "will be found sitting inside his house 'with head bowed under the imagined stare of the whole community.'"[40] Response to such a harangue is swift and severe. The shamed person averts his eyes, withdraws, or — in its extreme form — goes into hiding or exile.

Since the retaliatory fury and feelings of revenge can for the most part not be vented towards the group, it is turned inwards or inhibited, giving rise to various self-destructive acts. In a benign form (such as in *veumayiyi*[41]) the shamed person shames the shamer with an extravagant gift. In a more malignant form, the person becomes suicidal: Malinowski gives examples of people committing "flamboyant suicide" by jumping from palm trees after being shamed for transgressing a clan taboo.[42]

A particular form of shame is that which is felt for others who have been shamed and with whom one has identifications, especially in field-dependent subjects. The prototype of this reaction and its resolution is found in an account by Sack.[43] In former times it seems that when a woman had been shamed only her death could remove the shame. I interpret this as a pathway by which already-existing matricidal impulses can be discharged through a fantasy of "killing the shamed". This is confirmed by the fact that it was usually the woman's own son who led the killing party. It is my contention that this mechanism of "killing the shamed" in one of the most powerful, though deeply repressed, dynamics of the AIDS epidemic: that which is enacted in real murder in the tribal culture, becomes a more sublimated but nevertheless equally venomous outpouring of death wishes towards drug addicts and homosexuals. It is as if the shame of the offenders' misconduct were acutely felt by the rest of the group, so that only their elimination can remove the painful effects of the shame. These identifications are based on an unconscious resonance between the shamed ones and the rest of the group.

The epidemic of AIDS is an awesome demonstration of the power and destructiveness of so much concentrated shame. Moveover, in a particularly lethal combination, the harangue which was delivered by the New Right induced in homosexuals and drug addicts both guilt and shame. They were in effect told that they were bad (should feel shame for being homosexual or addicted), and that they had done wrong (were guilty of promiscuity and drug abuse). Since there was no effective action through which to get rid of the retaliatory rage, it was all turned in against themselves, causing a wave of shame- and guilt-induced depression in those who were most susceptible to the disapproval of the group (on the basis of individual psychological make-up). There have been reports of three people committing suicide after being diagnosed with AIDS in Sweden,[44] but none in the U.S.

DISTAL CAUSES

Group tensions can build up and be discharged over surprisingly long intervals. If we look at the statistics for the incidence of suicide in the U.S. during the twentieth century and compare that with the statistics for venereal disease, an interesting pattern emerges (Figures 5 & 6). Both of these reach a peak around a major war — peaks of suicide preceding and the peaks in venereal disease coinciding with or following the war — and an abnormally high plateau is reached by the curve for venereal disease during the mid-70s. From a group-psychological standpoint, we can make the interpretation that we are passing through the psychological equivalent of World War III, or that we are at its foothills. This can also be inferred from the apparent inverse relationship between world war and the incidence of epidemic hysteria, noted by Sirois.[45] The factor preventing a world war seems to me to be the invention of the nuclear bomb, since the powerful destructive force at man's disposal is far more than will ever be necessary for purposes of war. The enormous surplus of destructive power that may *not* be used (since total annihilation would exceed the ***sacrificial quota of war***) has led to an enormous curbing of fantasies of phallic aggressiveness. Everyone was made aware of these terrible atomic powers through the scare drills of the early 50s, which brought home to everyone how precarious our control over our group aggressions really is. (Interestingly enough, the age group most affected by AIDS, aged 30 - 39, were exposed to these drills during their early school years.) The nuclear freeze movement should be interpreted as a huge obsessive defense (reaction formation) against the use of these weapons.

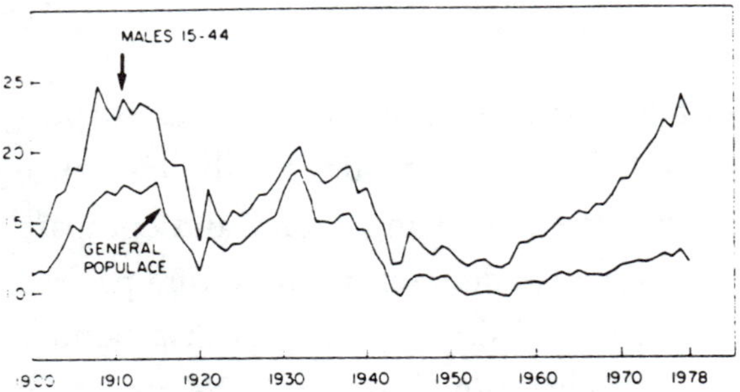

Figure 5
Incidence: Suicide (U.S., 1900-1978)[46]

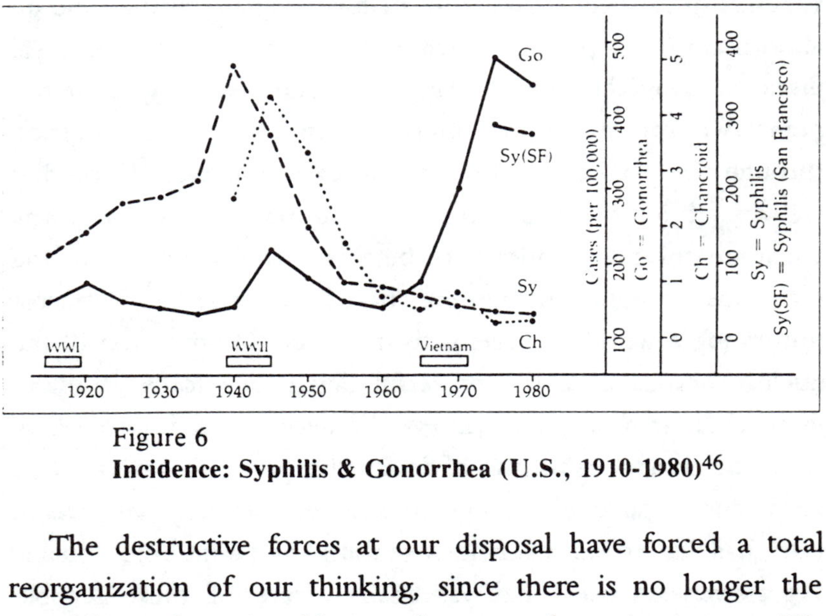

Figure 6
Incidence: Syphilis & Gonorrhea (U.S., 1910-1980)[46]

The destructive forces at our disposal have forced a total reorganization of our thinking, since there is no longer the possibility of a winnable war between the superpowers. We resort to fantasies, as in the case of World War II which is currently being touted, somewhat nostalgically, as "The Good War."[47] The pattern of warfare for both superpowers — China is ignored as a superpower for purposes of fantasy, since one has only two parents — has become one of war-by-proxy or displacement wars. Thus, Korea, Vietnam, and Central America for the U.S., and uprisings in the Eastern Bloc countries and

Afghanistan for the U.S.S.R. This curb on phallic- aggressive acting-out by the U.S. had led to widespread fears of being effeminate or impotent (fantasy: "We can't screw them, therefore we must be women.") As can be seen from the cartoons from the early part of the Reagan years (Figures 7 & 8), most of our phallic potency was injected into the Russians, who took on a frighteningly and humiliatingly masculine aspect, while America felt relatively impotent. These are, I think, the roots for the great need for "a winnable war" (between the superpowers) which is so apparent at this time. This curb on phallic-assertiveness created a feeling of gender dysphoria, which was then injected into the nations's homosexuals in fantasy. ("It's not we who feel weak and impotent, it's them.") This weakness and impotence "of America" was painfully conscious for all during the Carter years, and part of Reagan's mandate was to turn this around. After the invasion of Grenada the "balance of potency" was completely reversed (Figure 9), so that we felt proud again, or as the phrase went, "America [was] standing tall again."

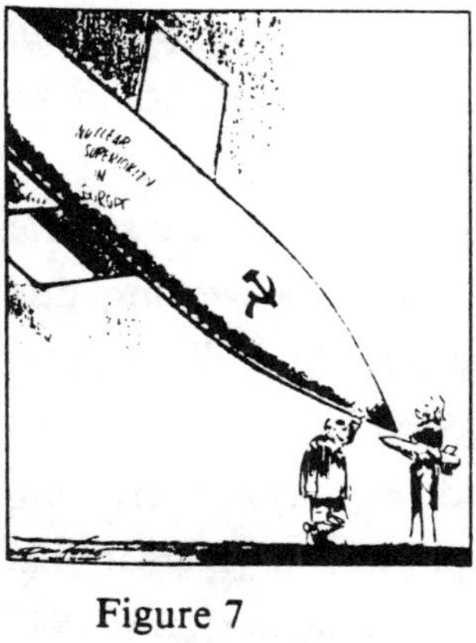

Figure 7
March, 1982

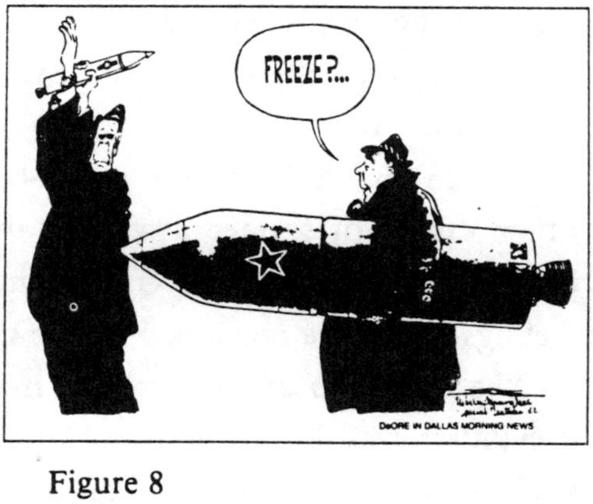

Figure 8
November, 1982

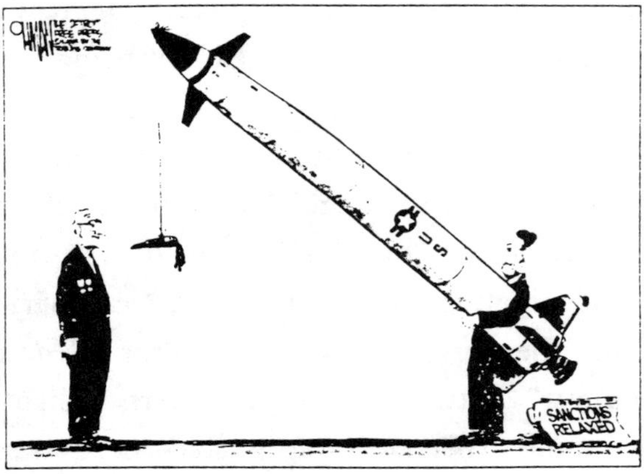

Figure 9
November, 1983

That these painful feelings of emasculation were intolerable to us, and that something drastic had to be done, was shown, and the solution implied by Alexander Haig's statement about the Falklands War (the "dress rehearsal" for the invasion of Grenada). He said: "Britain's action may have marked a turning point in a long and dangerous night of Western passivity",[48] after the thought of the Argentinian junta that "a Western democracy was too soft, too decadent to defend itself". After the Grenada invasion America exulted: "Thank God, we finally have a real man in the White House", and "U.S. soldier's boot prints in Grenada's soil have done more than the MX will do to make U.S. power credible." [49, 50]

But in the unconscious group-fantasies there were several other causes of gender dysphoria that rose in a swelling tide through the 60s and 70s, cresting in the 80s. And all of these feelings had to be contained by the homosexuals.

The invention of birth control methods far beyond anything previously available made possible an explosion of "recreational sex" (as opposed to an ideal of purely functional sex) and 1957 remains a watershed in the moral history of the world. The "sexual revolution", as it came to be known, created an enormous change in American family life, though this change was more dangerous in fantasy than in reality. The most distressing single factor was an overt sexual desire and a demand for orgasmic satisfaction on the part of women. That this was a threat can be seen in statements such as the following: "the incidence of male homosexuality has increased enormously — perhaps a hundred times — with the introduction of oral contraceptives."[51] In addition, such pleasurable sexuality — and so much of it — produced a massive build-up of guilt, which became more obvious as the 70s wore on, and they helped propel superego forces to center stage. Since the assumption of this anti-pleasure position, there has developed a sinister preoccupation in America with so-called "sexual compulsives" (i.e. those into whom we have projected our own sexual desires in fantasy), who are currently being "treated" in AA-type group sessions. It was into containers such as these that we poured both our own sexual wishes and to whom the punishment could then be applied. These groups have become, almost literally, whipping boys, as alternatively guilt and shame is induced. (A valuable critique of this method of "treatment" has been written by Stein[52] and Wedin,[53] for alcoholics and sexual compulsives respectively.) The homosexuals were chosen to be the model for "sexual compulsives" since their legendary sexual activity generated scorn, fear, and envy in the larger group. (During the years 1983-84 we also saw an increase in the TV coverage of the use of such groups, and on national television members of such groups were shown being humiliated and made to feel guilty — instead of having their intrapsychic conflicts solved.) The sexual revolution and the freeing up of heterosexual conduct was parallel to that in the homosexual community, but it was the latter that was chosen to represent those impulses we wished to disavow and punish. Indirect evidence for this comes from anecdotal reports that one of the major topics of conversation at meetings of scientists around AIDS is the sexual habits of the homosexuals.

The last and the most important of the distal causes of the epidemic, adding further unresolved tensions to the unconscious fire, is the effect of women's liberation on the group psychology of America. Srole and Fischer,[54] in a fascinating study of the long-term trends in mental health in women in the U.S., present persuasive evidence that something changed in the past 35 to 75 years. There was a distinct difference between the mental health of men and women when the Midtown Manhattan study was done in 1954, at which time women were more compromised than men. When a re-study was done in 1974 this difference had disappeared so that women were on par with men on all measures of mental health. My interpretation is that the child-rearing practices vis-à-vis girls improved decade by decade, giving rise to healthier and happier mothers in a positive feedback loop. It was this increase in psychological well-being, I posit (as per psychic primacy), that created a new generation of women with less passivity, less depression, more self-esteem — all of which gave rise to the women's movement.

The way these changes translated themselves into society at large can be read from the lifestyle changes in the U.S. since the 60s: women became more independent; there was an increase in the divorce and then the re-marriage rates (which signified that women were now less afraid of searching for better partners); women tended to become more assertive (demanding orgasm, and more often starting their own businesses); and entered the workforce in droves (with confident predictions that the pay gap will "narrow perceptibly" during the 80s). The effects were electrifying, similar to the earlier response to the suffragette movement. At that time suffrage was seen as dangerous "because it threatened the existence of separate spheres. If women voted, they will abandon the home and womanly virtues. The differences between the sexes would be obscured: men would lose their manhood and women would begin to act like men."[56] The response to the women's movement in unconscious fantasy was just as strong and fearful. The title page of an article in the *Ladies Home Journal* captures it neatly: next to a hand holding up a little flag that says, "Help!" stands the title, "The Hurting Husband", followed by "As more women try to change the scope of their marriages, more men suffer from 'liberation shock'."[56]

In *Dominus: A Woman Looks at Men's Lives* (1978), author Gittelson[57] traces the effect of the "new woman" on the consciousness (read: group-fantasy) of men. These quotations convey the tone: "the so-called feminist revolution has transformed the consciousness of American men more dramatically, more decisively — and perhaps more dangerously — than the consciousness of women."[58] And, "...the second storm of female liberation within this century was rising all around them."[59] Men "...yearned openly ... for the return of the 'unreconstructed female'."[60] She shows persuasively how the quest for orgasm, the changes in gender role definition, the new honesty about their feelings by dissatisfied housewives, and the solidarity of women turned male-female relationships upside-down. "A nation of little Wilburs ... cringed under Big Mama's broomstick, accepting the reprimand to their entire sex. 'It's the pussy-whipping of America.'"[61] This was one of the regressive positions men repaired to: passive-masochistic attachment to phallic mother. There were others: a flight into bisexuality ("the American flirtation with bisexuality expanded into a coast-to-coast affair"[62]); a flight into homosexuality, and its opposite, a flight into machismo. The men's movement consisted of a network of support groups across America. Anyone with a precarious sexual identity was massively threatened. Unacceptable sexual impulses that had been managed through control based on repression rather than by a more flexible control based on mastery, could not take the changes in sway, and started crumbling.

The new assertiveness in women kindled fears of impotence in men, and homosexual fears were exacerbated. Male bonding, a mounting "gay tide" and flirtations with homosexual experimentation were the regressive positions to which men retreated under the impact of this gender crisis. "Homosexuality is on the rise in today's society. And with the Women's Liberation Movement, more and more men are feeling threatened by women and choosing homosexual rather than heterosexual relationships."[61] These fears were the ones injected into the homosexuals, even though that solution in itself in turn generated other fears. The "state of pain between men and women" (as Gittelson's book cover puts it) resulted in fantasies of complete gender role reversal, with films about househusbands, about cross-dressing (*Victor/Victoria, Tootsie* and so on), a film about a pregnant man (*The Rabbit Test*, which is an example of the couvade syndrome) and by the early 80s there arose a preoccupation with androgynous rock stars.

Parallel to these changes in sexual morality came a greater acceptance of the use of various "recreational drugs" (marijuana, amyl nitrite, cocaine) as well as addictive drugs (narcotics). Folk heroes, like Timothy Leary, advocated hallucinogens and much of America went off, so to speak, on a huge cloud until and even beyond the anti-drug backlash of the mid-70s. The group solution to this problem was similar to that used for the gender dysphoria. In both cases containers had to be found who could contain all these pleasurable, but eminently punishable, wishes.

PROXIMAL CAUSES

A clue to the psychological transformation affecting America during the later 70s comes from what we know about a group trance.[64] Most extensively studied around hypnosis, the most germane quality of a trance is its self-limiting nature. Each person seems to be suggestible up to a point: once suggestions are made that conflict with the basic structure of the personality, the subject becomes increasingly agitated and ultimately wakes up out of the trance or, paradoxically, falls asleep. Multiplied by millions and spread out over 10 years, this seems to be a fair description of what happened to America in the late 70s. It was as if everyone had become involved in a pleasurable picnic since the 60s, and all of a sudden everyone simultaneously started waking up from the trance, shamefacedly scrambling for their clothes and hurrying home. This was the conservative clampdown.

By using several key indicators, it is possible to locate this change in unconsciously held attitudes more or less precisely. This is done by considering:

(a) retrospective assessments — "Future historians of the movement, in fact, may set the years of the sexual revolt at roughly 1965 to 1975."[65]

(b) Slips of the tongue, such as Robert Gallo's making the slip in 1984 that the epidemic of AIDS had started 9 years before.[66]

(c) The beginning of the clampdown on hardline drug abuse with the creation in 1975 of CENTAC 1 (a central tactical unit of the Drug Enforcement Administration) and 18 similar units since then.[67]

(d) A sudden swing in contributions of funds to political campaigns by large corporations — for example, a certain corporation that used to give 93% of its contributions to liberal causes in 1976 started giving only 17% to liberal causes in 1978, and this formed a trend.[68]

(e) The beginning of the clampdown on sexuality, which showed itself first through the backlash against "runaway gay liberation", spearheaded by the Anita Bryant campaign in Dade county, Florida in early 1977. This was followed by a series of "Anita Bryant Laws" in various states, the formation of Moral Majority, Inc., in 1978, Religious Roundtable in 1979, the phenomenal direct-mail missives on behalf of conservative causes by Richard Viguerie, and the apotheosis of conservatism with the election of Ronald Reagan in 1980.

(f) In the heterosexual sphere the equivalent was the concern over herpes, which was, as *Time* magazine put it, "Today's Scarlet Letter".[69] All of these changes ushered in a period of sadistic superego control and a turn away from pleasure. On the issue of "Sex in the '80s", we were informed by *Time* that "The Revolution Is Over",[70] and by *Newsweek* that "AIDS may mean the party is over."[71]

In terms of group process, such a period of clampdown (of which Prohibition and McCarthyism are earlier examples) consists of two components: a phase of internal sacrifice followed by a phase of external sacrifice. The latter usually takes the form of a war, and at this time the stage has been set for that in Central America.[72] Psychologically speaking, the phase of internal sacrifice is the result of a more advanced mode of group functioning, one which implies impulse control and the ability to delay gratification (and by not immediately going out and making war — such as is the norm for headhunters). It attempts to deal with certain group tensions by internal means rather than fighting them abroad or in others via projection. The phase of internal sacrifice started around 1975, intensifying by 1977, and was made into a formal doctrine in 1981 with the introduction of Reaganomics. (For an analysis of how this was done, see deMause's book, *Reagan's America*.[73]) The central tenet was one of the withdrawal of things that were seen as "too good": the withdrawal of permissiveness and the "end of the sexual revolution" in the sexual sphere; the withdrawal of food and services from women and children (from which emerged the guilty preoccupation with "hunger in America" during 1983; the withdrawal of permission for abortion; the withdrawal of permission for the use of drugs, culminating in Nancy Reagan's "War on Drugs" in the 80s; and a proliferation of bad feelings towards homosexuals, who had come to represent all the gender dysphoria that had accumulated over the previous two decades.

This conservative swing, as with all group-fantasy phenomena, affected the entire group, and all of America became more sober and conservative as the 80s wore on. In Berkeley, hotbed of protest in the 60s, students were now putting up posters of Reagan and saying, "I can definitely see us going to war."[74] Among homosexuals "the greatest growth of gay political activity is among Republican suburbanites."[75] In the psychological sphere there has been, all of a sudden, a spate of anti-Freudian or anti-shrink books.[76] In television the half-hour sitcom made, during the 1983-84 season, its "worst showing in 30 years; not a single sitcom that ran all season was ranked among the top ten" as contrasted with the 1974-75 season, when 7 did.[77] Action programs like "The A-Team" and others responded to our new warlike mood and did well.

In the accompanying graph (Figure 10) I have indicated the relationship between this conservative swing and the incidence of AIDS, as it relates to real and perceived threats against homosexuals. It is possible to draw up similar graphs for drug abuse and the turn of popular opinion against that. (As in the rest of the paper I will concentrate on the group dynamics as it pertains to the homosexuals, and refer to the others only briefly and in passing.) It must be kept in mind that these constitute conscious factors, which, in their appearance, were preceded by an "incubation period", as the unconscious impulses slowly percolated through to consciousness.

Above the line I depict the incidence of AIDS for the U.S. as a whole, and that of amebiasis for San Francisco. Below the line are listed those incidents that seemed to attain symbolic significance (based on attention paid to them in the homosexual periodicals and on psychohistorical interpretation). (For example, the Briggs-sponsored Proposition 6 — which would have barred homosexuals from teaching in public schools — was defeated in a referendum; yet, since it was concrete evidence of the strength of the clampdown, it is included.) As can be seen, the incidence of amebiasis begins to rise to epidemic levels immediately after the postulated swing in unconscious attitude, and that of AIDS starts to climb about 2 to 4 years after the clampdown became "official" through the campaign of Anita Bryant. (In the medical paper I advance the hypothesis that this lag period depends on the turnaround time for the development of T-helper cells.) The formal introduction of Reaganomics in 1981 coincides with the first clinical descriptions of AIDS, thus confirming the unconscious

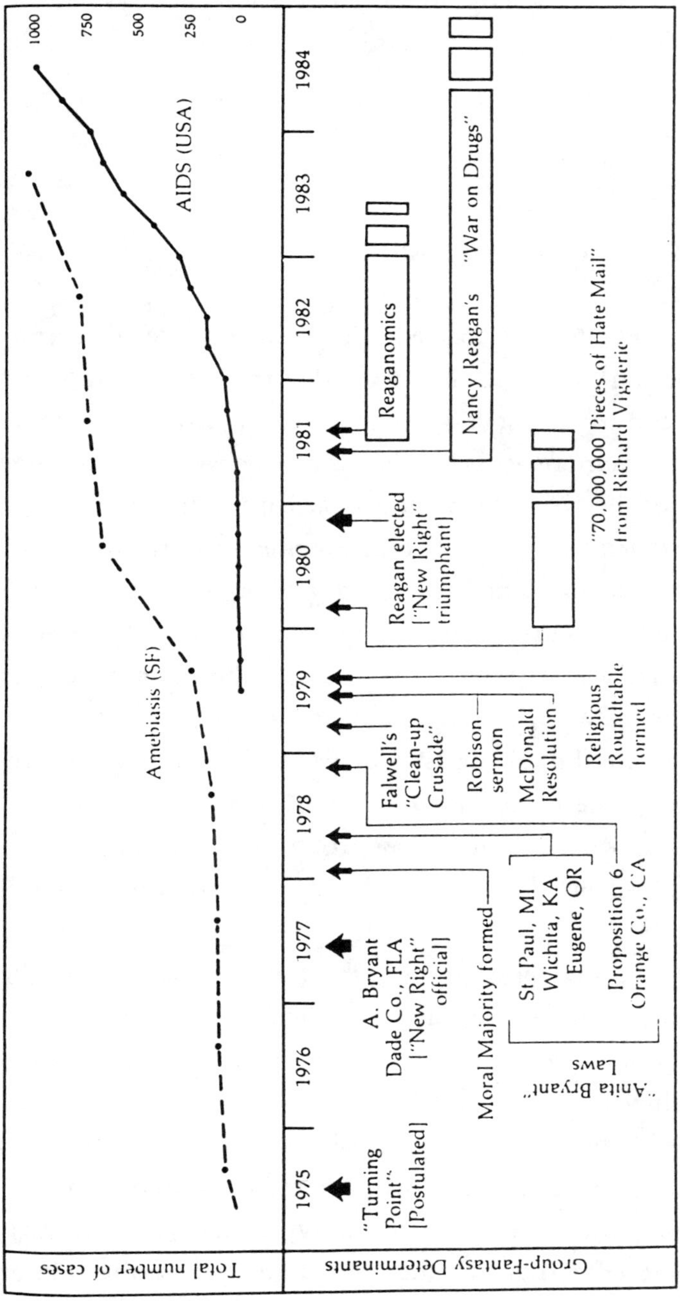

Figure 10
Conservative Clampdown in U.S. *versus* Incidence of AIDS (U.S.) & Amebiasis (S.F.)

group-fantasies, and setting up the positive feedback system that has propelled the epidemic forward ever since.

HISTORY OF AN EPIDEMIC

I. Line-up for the clash

Groups, in Slater's celebrated phrase, have a "peculiar, crab-like locomotion", by which he meant that they move slowly and strangely, and often obliquely to or away from the point. Nowhere is this more apparent than in the behavior of the three subgroups of the U.S. who came to participate in the origins of the AIDS epidemic. I would like to examine, in turn, the major outlines of what happened to the "gay rights movement" after 1973-74, and the contribution by the homosexuals to the "war of morality" that was to follow; the rise and the move to center stage of the New Right, especially the contribution that the formation of the Moral Majority and the anti-gay rights movement made to the group-fantasy origins of AIDS; and finally, I will take a look at the largest subgroup of Americans, the so-called "silent majority" and what part they played in this clash of ideologies.

The first of the three groups, the homosexuals, essentially turned their aggression inward (by somatizing tensions) and played the role of the masochistic partner in the scapegoating ritual which was to follow. This position was dictated by an "internalized homophobia" (a total misnomer for "identifications with their aggressors and those who wished them to disappear"), and is similar to that taken by all martyred scapegoats through the ages. The second group, the New Right, played the role of sadist in this scapegoating battle, slinging death threats in the direction of the homosexuals with an absence of empathy and full of righteousness. The third group, the silent majority of Americans, at first took little notice. Everyone was swinging to the right, and by 1981 Goldwater could say, "It's a wonderful feeling to be a conservative these days", since such a position had the full support of the group-fantasy. Around Reagan's election they started playing up the role of the New Right, for example, by television and media coverage exceeding the extent to which the general public subscribed to their notions. A Gallup poll taken in 1980 on this issue (the definition of a group-fantasy issue in America) showed that less than 50 percent of Americans knew about the Moral Majority, that only 23 percent saw themselves as belonging to the "New Christian Right" and only 8 percent approved of the goals of the Moral Majority.[78] This behavior by mainstream America towards the New Right is typical for behavior shown towards delegate groups: these groups quietly practise their own, usually somewhat fanatical, group-fantasies in the wings until they are needed by the majority. They are then called to center stage, and quietly nudged (like an adolescent in a family) into acting out some of the conflicted needs of the group, after which they are "discarded".

II. Anlagen for Heroic Suicide

I do not review here the history of the "gay rights movement", and refer the reader elsewhere for excellent overviews.[79] Suffice it to say that a wave of excited self-revelation and self-discovery, followed by a "new boldness", spread through the homosexual community from 1969 onwards (after a group of homosexuals attacked police who were raiding the Stonewall bar in New York City). By 1973-74 two rather profound changes were to take place in the official standing of homosexuality in America. The psychiatrists (father imagoes onto whom homosexuals have traditionally displaced their rage and hatred, a position that has since been reserved for "Freudian analysts") reversed themselves as a group in 1973 and declared that homosexuality *per se* was no longer considered to be a psychiatric disorder. In 1974 the American Psychological Association followed suit. Throughout the early 70s many states were re-writing their criminal codes, and by 1976 about half of the United States had revoked their sodomy statutes. On this issue there was hearty criticism from conservatives such as Reagan, who said in 1976, "I would have vetoed it. You can make immorality legal but you cannot make it moral."[80] During 1976 the pace of anti-discrimination laws being passed slowed down to a considerable extent.

Meanwhile homosexuals all over America were coming out of the closet (from Air Force Sergeants to professional football players), swept along in the euphoria of their new-found assertiveness and the acceptance which they read in the recognition by the two major psychological blocs: "Come out, come out...." they exulted, "gay people are not invisible anymore...."[81] It is my impression that many people who came out were ill-prepared for what was to follow once they were to meet prejudice face-to-face, since few had sufficiently worked-through the issues of shame and guilt involved. More important, many people in mainstream America were just as ill-prepared for it, as became clear in retrospect. The sense of freedom (from external constraints) was heady, and a large sector of the homosexual community were "living in a very fast trajectory indeed, at a high velocity fueled by late nights and early mornings, of dancing for hours without a break, of taking drugs and having sex with a lot of very handsome, strong, powerful, wonderful men."[82] In clinical experience, sudden freedom before a person has adequately been prepared is rarely tolerated well, since there is not always sufficient ego structure to cope with it. Fall-back positions then include: rigid self-control through denial of too much pleasure or, as a regressive position, submission to external controls. Before this liberation into mania, external controls had been built into the system, so that excesses of lifestyle as were later described were rare, and self-limiting.

On the heels of the sexual revolution followed an epidemic of venereal disease, with an incidence that shot sky-high during the 60s and remained high throughout the 70s. In the mid-70s the term "gay bowel syndrome" was coined for the plethora of illnesses encountered by proctologists. Significantly, as I had alluded to about the penumbral syndrome of AIDS, the incidence of amebiasis abruptly took off in 1975, with a dramatic increase over the previous year. Since no overt change in sexual habits took place in 1974 (such as a sudden introduction of anilingus), we have to look for alternative explanations. I posit that a sudden change took place in the unconscious group-fantasies of the homosexuals at that moment, a covert event which was translated into psychosomatic symptoms and augured in the coming epidemic. "How long, [they] began to wonder, could this marvelous pleasure last?"[82] My supposition is that a build-up of guilt had taken place, based on the new lifestyle, and that it showed itself in this way at first. An additional clue can be read from an advertisement that ran in *The Advocate* (the most important homosexual newspaper at that time), for about 2 years on and off, starting in 1975. It was an ad for the GSF (Gay Social Forum), and ran as its eye-catcher the line, "The Only Happy Homosexual Is A Dead One."[83] This was carefully rationalized as a statement by the "enemy", and went on to speak of "a lifetime of suicide". I interpret this as the first sign of the massive build-up of unconscious guilt over such sexual abandon, a particularly difficult demon to placate and one which was to demand many sacrifices in times ahead.

A recent example of the same submissive, sacrificial attitude is found in an advertisement for the Metropolitan Community Church (which is a congregation of homosexuals).[84] The MCC is one of the favorite targets of Jerry Falwell, and the ad quotes him as preaching on the "Old Time Gospel Hour": "Thank God this vile and satanic system will one day be utterly annihilated and there will be a celebration in heaven." The MCC's response to this is a gentle: "No Jerry, that's not what the Metropolitan Community Church is like because: We are a caring, loving group of people. We have created a 60-minute television documentary to confront those kind of lies...." This is an attitude identical to that of Jews trying to convince Nazis that they were in fact quite patriotic and German, and equally futile. (For an analysis of the group dynamics of the masochistic partner in a sado-masochistic ritual on the historical stage, I refer the reader to Stein.)[85] Clinically and historically one finds that this type of meekness invites further sadistic onslaught, so that the system becomes self-perpetuating.

Whatever death wishes the homosexuals may have been unconsciously entertaining towards themselves in 1975, they were just that: wishes. Soon, however, as they were continuing to be projected into the "enemy out there", they found an object to stick to, which escalated the seriousness. As long as one perceived threats where there are none, all is vaguely well. When someone responds to that perceived threat and starts to really threaten you, it sets up a process of resonance, making one's greatest fear become very real and inducing dread. This is, I think, what happened around the time of that crucial switch in the mid-70s. By July 1976 the United Federation of Teachers went on record against gay rights.[86] By early 1977 the homosexual press started reporting that students on campuses were wearing T-shirts saying: "Bury a Fairy" or "Do the world a favor — Shoot a Faggot."[87] The process of liberalization, though slowed down, continued. Dade county, Florida had passed a gay rights ordinance in February — the first major city in the previous year. There had been active campaigning by the homosexuals since the previous November, and it was the first victory by a "gay political machine" of its kind. And here, in the spring of 1977, the stage was set for the clampdown-to-come.

III. The New Right Shows Its Fist

Enter Anita Bryant, an unhappy singer who identifies herself with "Deborah in the Bible whom God chose in a period of spiritual depravity when male leaders weren't what they should be...."[88] Her marriage of many years' standing unhappy, unfulfilling and on the brink of divorce, she feels herself drawn to lead the counterrevolution. She leads the attack on gay rights, and founds at first "Save Our children (From Homosexuals), Inc." and later "Anita Bryant Ministries". The popularity of this cause is evident in the more than $2 million contributed by 400,000 people within the first 10 months.[89] In her book, *The Anita Bryant Story* — subtitled: *The Survival of our Nation's Families and the Threat of Militant Homosexuality* — she outlines the major issues: "The women's liberation programs ... have weakened family ties ... single men are the chief source of crime and social disruption

... marriage is essential to male socialization...."[90] The gay rights movement is an "escape from sexual responsibilities and its display a threat to millions of young men who have precarious masculine identities."[91] That all of this would lead to a sacrificial ritual in which people would actually have to die, is clear from statements such as: "they were *sacrificially* committing themselves to whatever was necessary to save our children" (my emphasis)[93] and "I'm not out with a Bible in one hand and a sword in the other" (negation).[94] She correctly foresaw that "a repeal [of the gay rights ordinance] would send a tidal wave of repression all across the country."[95] She quoted a Dr. Lindsell: "If he [the homosexual] does not repent, he is doomed...."[96] A commingling of her personal and the group's fears are revealed in: "...as the more liberal life-styles come into the open, divorce rates soar, leaving the debris of human tragedy behind to suffer. The debris? Our children."[97]

As the campaign heated up in Dade county, homosexuals realized exactly what was going on, and became appropriately scared. Their most outstanding response to this threat, however, was also the most self-destructive: they started wearing little pink triangles, like those that had been issued to homosexuals under the Third Reich, saying, in effect, "We are your willing sacrificial victims."[98] Bumper stickers in Dade county started to sport overt death wishes: "KILL A QUEER FOR CHRIST."[99]

When the vote was tallied, victory was in the hands of Bryant and the New Right. She flashed a "dazzling smile of triumph. The 'normal majority' have said, 'Enough! Enough! Enough!'"[100] It was obvious to Sergeant Leonard Matlovitch (a former Vietnam War Hero who had deliberately provoked a discharge from the Air Force in 1975 by informing his superior officer that he was gay) that a wave of repression was indeed going to follow, as well as the sacrificial events that Bryant had prophetically foretold. He warned that "Stormy times are ahead. I fear repression. *Some gays are going to have to be prepared to make sacrifices — even die.*" (my emphasis).[101]

Those were the first pieces of the puzzle: the delivery of the harangue was underway. In contrast to the simple recitation in the quiet of the Papuan night, this harangue was to be delivered in a stream of bitter fragments scattered across all the media and the mail for the next few years.[102] The picture that emerges from the examples of direct-mail solicitations I have seen shows a distorted, overblown image of a militant, marching cadre of homosexuals and America about to be engulfed by Sodom and Gomorrah. Against this "fearsome foe" the New Right mobilized all their forces. In his "Declaration of War",[103] Falwell writes that "the Old Time Gospel Hour hereby declares war against the evils threatening America during the 1980s ... this shall be a Holy War, not a war with guns and bullets ... lead an army of Christian soldiers into the war against evil" (Figure 11). The Evils to be fought against are abortion, the murder of innocent babies, and homosexuality as the cause of the deterioration of home and family. He vows in another letter to "continue to expose the sin of homosexuality.... I believe that the massive homosexual revolution is always a symptom of a nation coming under the judgment of God.... *The homosexuals are on the march in this country.*"[104] Behind the fear of homosexuals was a conspiracy: "the drive for homosexual rights ... [is] just a fraction of a master plan to destroy everything that is good and moral here in America", said another.[105]

It is impossible to estimate the numbers of letters and appeals such as these that went out in the U.S. mail: the *Moral Majority Report* goes out to 840,000 homes per month, and there is no way

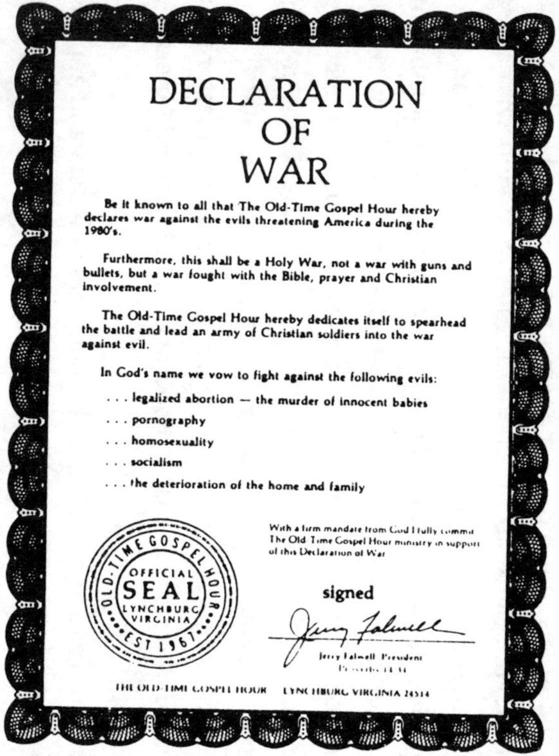

DECLARATION
OF
WAR

Be it known to all that The Old-Time Gospel Hour hereby declares war against the evils threatening America during the 1980's.

Furthermore, this shall be a Holy War, not a war with guns and bullets, but a war fought with the Bible, prayer and Christian involvement.

The Old-Time Gospel Hour hereby dedicates itself to spearhead the battle and lead an army of Christian soldiers into the war against evil.

In God's name we vow to fight against the following evils:

. . . legalized abortion — the murder of innocent babies

. . . pornography

. . . homosexuality

. . . socialism

. . . the deterioration of the home and family

With a firm mandate from God I fully commit The Old-Time Gospel Hour ministry in support of this Declaration of War

OLD-TIME GOSPEL HOUR OFFICIAL SEAL LYNCHBURG VIRGINIA EST 1967

signed

Jerry Falwell

Jerry Falwell, President

THE OLD-TIME GOSPEL HOUR LYNCHBURG VIRGINIA 24514

Figure 11
The Harangue
against Homosexuals
A: Sadistic Partners

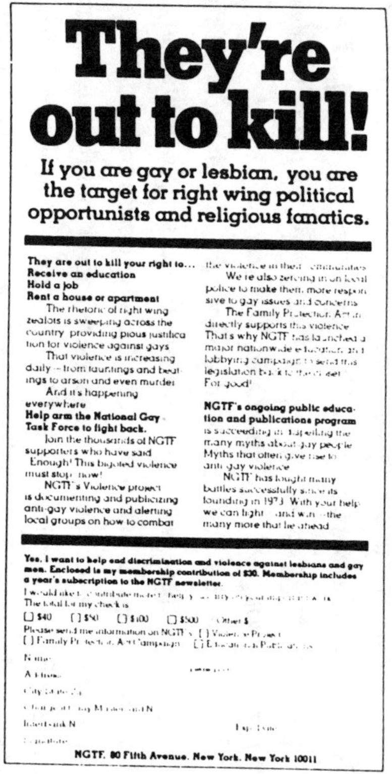

They're out to kill!

If you are gay or lesbian, you are the target for right wing political opportunists and religious fanatics.

They are out to kill your right to...
Receive an education
Hold a job
Rent a house or apartment

The rhetoric of right wing zealots is sweeping across the country providing pious justification for violence against gays.

That violence is increasing daily — from tauntings and beatings to arson and even murder.

And it's happening everywhere.

Help arm the National Gay Task Force to fight back.

Join the thousands of NGTF supporters who have said Enough! This bigoted violence must stop now!

NGTF's Violence project is documenting and publicizing anti-gay violence and alerting local groups on how to combat the violence in their communities.

We're also zeroing in on local police to make them more responsive to gay issues and concerns.

The Family Protection Act directly supports this violence. That's why NGTF has launched a major nationwide education and lobbying campaign to send this legislation back to the closet. For good!

NGTF's ongoing public education and publications program is succeeding in dispelling the many myths about gay people. Myths that often give rise to anti-gay violence.

NGTF has fought many battles successfully since its founding in 1973. With your help we can fight — and win — the many more that lie ahead.

Yes, I want to help end discrimination and violence against lesbians and gay men. Enclosed is my membership contribution of $30. Membership includes a year's subscription to the NGTF newsletter.

The total for my check is

[ ] $40 [ ] $50 [ ] $100 [ ] $500 Other $

Please send me information on NGTF's [ ] Violence Project [ ] Family Protection Act Campaign [ ] Educational Publications

Name

Address

City State Zip

Interbank N

Signature

NGTF, 80 Fifth Avenue, New York, New York 10011

Figure 12
The Harangue
against Homosexuals
B: Masochistic Partners

of estimating the volume of mail sent out by Richard Viguerie's direct-mail empire.[106] That the Moral Majority knew that they were engaged in a witch hunt ("Holy War") was evident from statements made at training seminars such as, "We're here to learn how to burn witches and everything else the press says we're about."[107] Sentiments were expressed blatantly: "I know what you and I feel about these queers, these fairies. We wish we could get in our cars and run them down while they march...."[108] Another: "I agree with capital punishment and I believe that homosexuality ... could be coupled with murder and other sins.... It would be the government that sits upon this land who will be executing the homosexuals."[109] And: "The cure to cancer is not to ignore it — remove it."

Then there were "the recent efforts of the so-called 'American Party for Manhood' to bring back capital punishment for homosexuals."[110] Death wishes were also issued by the church: "I was told by a sincere Christian counselor that it would be 'better' to 'repent and die', even if I had to kill myself, than to go on living and relating to others as a homosexual."[111] These are quotes from a radio preacher: "Sodom and Gomorrah were turned into ashes as an example of how God feels about being gay...." and "God dropped an atomic bomb on Sodom and Gomorrah because they were perverts!"[112] Some said, "A very good case can be made out that the homosexual is the modern equivalent of the leper" and that "the children of Israel were commanded by God to stone to death homosexuals (Lev. 20:13), a severe treatment intended to keep them from becoming contagious."[113] Here we are on the threshold of the poison fantasies of the epidemic proper. Anita Bryant was intuitively homing in on another of the core fantasies (though at this time still with an admixture of cannibalism) when she said that God does not like homosexuals because "the male homosexual eats another man's sperm. Sperm is the most concentrated form of blood. The homosexual is eating life."[114]

Put together succinctly, this whole catalogue of threats delivered into the public arena (starting with Bryant's campaign materials which contained a paper entitled, "Why Certain Sexual Deviations Are Punishable By Death") points to one end, which is "Death to the Homosexuals." And this was indeed the message they picked up. Full-page advertisements such as the one depicted here (Figure 12) have been run since the AIDS epidemic started.[115] It shows how the death threats and the clampdown have been internalized: gone was the gallows humor of "The only happy homosexual is a dead one."

A similar harangue was delivered to the drug addicts of the U.S. with, as is my thesis, identical results. In Figure 13 I have collated newspaper headlines from the past 4 years. Not surprisingly there has been an epidemic of heroin-related deaths in the Washington, D.C. area for the past 4 years, with a death rate higher than any previously reported in the literature.[116] These harangues, with their severe public shaming of these two groups for irrational reasons, were the factors that intensified whatever change had taken place in 1975, and were thus the direct precipitants of the AIDS epidemic.

BEYOND EPIDEMIC AIMS

The cure for an epidemic of hysteria is extremely simple. Once identified as such, all one has to do is to publicly announce it to be an epidemic of "mass hysteria", after which the epidemic resolves itself in a very short space of time.

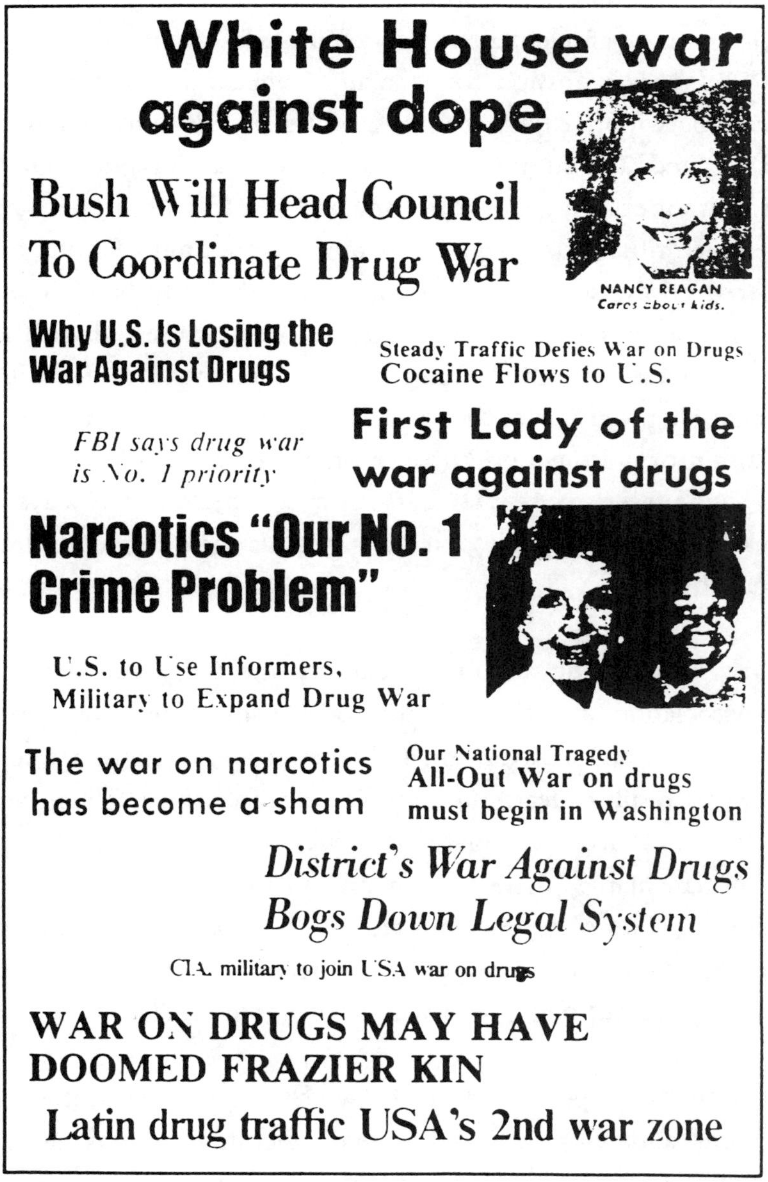

White House war against dope

Bush Will Head Council To Coordinate Drug War

NANCY REAGAN
Cares about kids.

Why U.S. Is Losing the War Against Drugs

Steady Traffic Defies War on Drugs
Cocaine Flows to U.S.

FBI says drug war is No. 1 priority

First Lady of the war against drugs

Narcotics "Our No. 1 Crime Problem"

U.S. to Use Informers, Military to Expand Drug War

The war on narcotics has become a sham

Our National Tragedy
All-Out War on drugs must begin in Washington

District's War Against Drugs Bogs Down Legal System

CIA, military to join USA war on drugs

WAR ON DRUGS MAY HAVE DOOMED FRAZIER KIN

Latin drug traffic USA's 2nd war zone

Figure 13
The Harangue against Drug Addicts

In an outbreak of psychosomatic symptoms due to a suspected poison gas at an elementary school in Dade County, Florida (in 1976)[117], it was possible for Nitzkin to effectively terminate the epidemic within a time span of 2 hours and 10 minutes after it was started. The rumor that a gas leak was causing girls to faint (fantasy of poison gas) had started and spread within one hour, by which time most major news media from South Florida had arrived on the scene. By announcing that the disturbance was a mass hysteria and that there were no toxic causes, all further attacks were prevented and the school returned to its usual functioning. During the Koro epidemic in Singapore in 1967 a delusion of poisoned pork (based on recent vaccinations of pigs for swine fever) caused 469 persons over a period of 10 days to seek help in great panic that their genitals were retracting into their bodies.

> "After public announcements by the Singapore Medical Association and the Ministry of Health were given wide exposure on television and in the newspapers stating that koro was a result of fear, not a physical disease with fatalities, and that meat from inoculated pigs was completely harmless to human beings, there was an immediate decline in the incidence of koro. Several days after these public announcements there were only a few cases reported, and within a month koro was not being reported in Singapore at all."[118]

There are two mechanisms by which this resolution may be brought about: (a) the old analytic dictum of "making the unconscious conscious", whereby the unconscious fantasies are robbed of their powerful sway over the conscious mind; and (b) the person who takes control and makes the announcement serves to reassure the affected cases that rationality and sanity will prevail. The officials act as containers for the anxieties of the group.

Nitzkin (as did Kerckhoff)[119] outlines how the medical response to such an epidemic is a powerful and determining factor in its outcome. In a similar epidemic of koro in Thailand, the medical authorities did not take the same calm, reassuring stance as they did in Singapore — with the result that the epidemic dragged on for (unnecessary) months.[120] To respond in a way that confirms the group delusion — to pull out all the medical stops with blood tests and hospitalizations, and the general "epidemic hoopla" of heightened emotions and excited poison hunters — is to perpetuate the epidemic. (This in no way precludes consideration of toxic causes when appropriate.) In fact, Nitzkin reports:

> In several of these outbreaks, the diagnosis was strongly suspected early in the outbreak but not acted upon because the investigators apparently believed that such a diagnosis could not be announced or acted upon until all other diagnoses had been "completely ruled out".[121]

This means that epidemic hysteria, in those few cases where it is at all considered, usually remains an exclusion diagnosis rather than a positive gestalt that can be identified on its own criteria (bias against psychological diagnoses). Apart from a lack of knowledge about this entity (quite prevalent since so few of the textbooks carry the information and it is not included in the current diagnostic manual of American psychiatry, the DSM-III), another factor obscures the picture. It seems to me that the crucial, inhibiting factor is the extent to which the medical examiner comes to share the belief in the poison threat. If the medical professionals cannot disentangle themselves from this belief, they will be powerless to terminate the epidemic, and it will have to wind down on its own.

If AIDS is indeed found to be an epidemic of depression with psychogenically reduced cell-mediated immunity, it follows from my argument that a simple announcement to this effect will have the desired therapeutic result. However, all therapeutic efforts so far have been applied to short epidemics (2 hours and 10 minutes in Dade County, and 10 days in Singapore). The time needed for a resolution ought therefore to be proportionately longer, and about 2 to 4 years (the turnaround time for the development of the T-helper cells and enough time to slough off the belief in poison sperm and blood) ought to be a minimum. This time period may be shortened by psychotherapy, adjunctive therapies and a rational stance from officials in whom the public places faith.

My sense, however, is that an announcement that any particular epidemic is an example of epidemic hysteria will be met with resistance among those who subscribe to the group delusion, and for whom the epidemic is a golden solution to unconscious conflicts. The larger the number of people subscribing to the delusion, the stronger I would expect the resistance to be to such an announcement (magnification effect of the group). Since it would also give rise to power struggles among people over whose beliefs are stronger or more accurate, such an announcement will have to come from someone held in very high esteem for having impeccable scientific credibility. In the AIDS epidemic, with the entire Western world sharing a belief that AIDS is caused by promiscuity and two fluids containing a virus, one should expect a truly monumental outpouring of hatred and resistance to such an announcement.

So strongly can a fantasy press upon the minds of scientists and laymen alike that evidence is frequently misinterpreted in order to fit in with more comfortable notions, or, as was pathetically and poignantly done in the case of a phantom epidemic of gonorrhea in a primary school, the wished-for evidence can even be hallucinated.[122] Viruses have been found in patients with AIDS and related conditions in 1983-84. I remain skeptical about their role in the etiology of AIDS, since their discovery generated immoderate enthusiasm and was felt to vindicate all the fantasies of poison sperm, poison blood and dangerous promiscuity. And because a reasonable hypothesis with sufficient explanatory power to account for virtually all of the known facts of the epidemic can be formulated without invoking them.

At this point the only attempts at cure from the lay public have been along the line of the "epidemic aims" (such as reducing sexual activity and numbers of sexual partners, and the widespread apotropaic ritual of "safe sex"). As with other epidemics which have a psychological component, there is a certain blindness to many aspects of the epidemic in one's midst, due to the group trance. I suspect it will be found, as with epidemics of heroin abuse, "that a community's awareness ... often comes only after the epidemic has peaked and is already on the decline."[123] Once the peak has been passed (i.e. when the unconscious driving forces are on the decline) it becomes easier to wake up out of the trance. One can only hope, for the sake of the 2,500 people in the United States living with a diagnosis of AIDS, and the 90-odd who are newly diagnosed each week, that we wake up from the trance, and soon.

REFERENCES

I would like to thank Lloyd deMause and David Reisel, without whose support and inspiration this essay would not have been possible.

1. Major recent reviews are: Francois Sirois, "Epidemic Hysteria", *Acta Psychiatrica Scandinavica*, 1974; Suppl. 252, 1-45. R.E. Markush, "Mental Epidemics: A Review of the Old to Prepare for the New", *Public Health Reviews*, 1973; 2: 353-442. George Mora, "An Historical and Socio-psychiatric Appraisal of Tarantism and its Importance in the Tradition of Psychotherapy of Mental Disorders", *Bulletin of the History of Medicine*, 1962; 36: 13-44. One book has been devoted in its entirely to the subject: *Mass Psychogenic Illness: A Social Psychological Analysis*, edited by Michael J. Colligan, James W. Pennebaker & Lawrence R. Murphy (Hillside, NJ: Lawrence Erlbaum, 1982).

2. Markush, *loc. cit.*, p. 396, 404.

3. Alan C. Kerckhoff & Kurt W. Back, *The June Bug: A Study of Hysterical Contagion* (New York: Appleton-Century-Crofts, 1968). The same epidemic was also reported in: Francis P. Champion *et al.*, "Mass Hysteria Associated with Insect Bites", *J. So. Carolina Med. Assn.*, 1963; 59:351-53.

4. Francois Sirois, "Perspectives on Epidemic Hysteria" in Colligan *et al.*, *op. cit.*, pp. 217-236.

5. Sirois, *ibid.*, p. 231.

6. Sirois, *ibid.*, p. 232.

7. John Frosch, *The Psychotic Process* (New York: International Universities Press, 1983), pp. 417-418, 140-149.

8. Silvano Arieti, "Introductory Notes on the Psychoanalytic Therapy of Schizophrenics", in *Psychotherapy of the Psychoses*, ed. A. Burton (New York: Basic Books, 1961).

9. H. Rosenfeld, "Note on the psychopathology of confusional states in chronic schizophrenia", *Int. J. Psycho-Anal.*, 1950; 31:132-137.

10. Melitta Sperling, *Psychosomatic Disorders in Childhood* (New York: Jason Aronson, 1978).

11. Elizabeth B. Weller & Ronald A. Weller, "Case Report of Conversion Symptom Associated with Major Depressive Disorder in a Child", *Am. J. Psychiatry*, 1983; 140: 1079-1080.

12. Norman Cohn, *Warrant for Genocide* (New York: Harper & Row, 1966), pp. 32, 186-7, 204 and especially 261-263.

13. Jean Fogo Russell, "Tarantism", *Medical History*, 1979; 23: 404-425, p. 408.

14. Jean Fogo Russell, "Dancing Mania", in *Festschrift for Kenneth Fitzpatrick Russell* (Melbourne: Queensberry Hill Press, 1978), p. 8.

15. B.H. Kagwa, "The problem of mass hysteria in East Africa", *East African Med. J.*, 1964; 41: 560-566.

16. Lyle Koehler, *A Search for Power: The "Weaker Sex" in Seventeenth-Century New England* (Urbana: University of Illinois Press, 1980), p. 391, quoted from: Robert Cales, *More Wonders of the Invisible World* (London: 1700), p. 355.

17. James W. Edwards, "Semen Anxiety in South Asian Cultures: Cultural and Transcultural Significance", *Med. Anthropol.*, 1983; 7: 51-67.

18. W. Jilek & L. Jilek-Aall, "A Koro Epidemic in Thailand", *Transcultural Psychiatr. Res.*, 1977; 15: 57-58.

19. W.H. Phoon, "Outbreaks of Mass Hysteria at Workplaces in Singapore: some Patterns and Modes of Presentation", in Colligan *et al., op.cit.*, p. 24. Similarly dramatic is the cleavage in the Thai koro epidemic where, though they form 10 percent of the population, not one case was reported among the Chinese: Sangun Suwanlert & Donald Coates, "Epidemic koro in Thailand — Clinical and Social Aspects", *Transcult. Psychiatr. Res*, 1978; 16: 64-66.

20. Harry D. Eastwell, "Psychological Disorders Among the Australian Aboriginals", in *Extraordinary Disorders of Human Behavior*, ed. Claude T.H. Friedmann & Robert A. Faguet (New York: Plenum, 1982), p. 237.

21. Donald W. Johnson, "The 'Phantom Anesthetist' of Mattoon: A Field Study of Mass Hysteria", *J. Abnorm. Soc. Psychol.*, 1943; 40: 175-186.

22. *The Lancet*, 1983; 8: 51.

23. *The Washington Post*, March 17, 1983, p. A8. This was at first known as the "voodoo connection". *Daily News*, February 28, 1983, p. 33.

24. *The Advocate*, March 20, 1984, p. 21.

25. *Newsweek*, May 7, 1984, p. 101.

26. Casper G. Schmidt, "AIDS Jokes; or, *Schadenfreude* Around an Epidemic", *Maledicta*, 1984; 8: *in press.*

27. Saul Nathaniel Brody, *The Disease of the Soul: Leprosy in Medieval Literature* (Ithaca: Cornell University Press, 1974), pp. 138-9.

28 *Ibid.*, p. 55.

29 *Ibid.*, p. 54.

30. *Ibid.*, p. 54.

31. *Ibid.*, p. 54.

32. Kurt W. Back, "Epidemiology versus Cartesian Dualism", *Soc. Sci. & Med.*, 1971; 5: 461-468.

33. J. Angst, "Masked Depression viewed from the cross-cultural standpoint", in *Masked Depression*, ed. P. Kielholz (Bern: Hans Huber Publishers, 1973, pp. 269-274.

34. Lloyd deMause, "The Evolution of Childhood", in *Foundations of Psychohistory* (New York: Creative Roots, 1982), pp. 1-83.

35. S.F. Maier & M.E. P. Seligman, "Learned Helplessness: Theory and Evidence", *J. Exp. Psychol.*, 1976; 105: 3-46.

36. Steven F. Maier, "Learned Helplessness, Depression, Analgesia, and Endogenous Opiates", *Psychopharm. Bull.*, 1983; 19: 531-536.

37. Helen Block Lewis, *Shame and Guilt in Neurosis* (New York: International Universities Press, 1971), pp. 83-91.

38. *Ibid.*, p. 275, pp. 311-316.

39. G. Piers & M. B. Singer, *Shame and Guilt: A Psychoanalytic and a Cultural Study* (New York: Norton, 1953), p. 29.

40. A.L. Epstein, *The Experience of Shame in Melanesia* (Royal Anthropological Institute of Great Britain and Ireland: Occasional Paper No. 40, 1984) (Atlantic Highlands, N.J. Humanities Press, distributors), p. 12.

41. *Ibid.*, p. 13.

42. Bronislav Malinowski, *Crime and Custom in Savage Society* (London: Routledge & Kegan Paul, 1926).

43. P. Sack, "The range of traditional Tolai remedies", in *Contention and Dispute: Aspects of Law and Social Control in Melanesia*, ed. A.L. Epstein (Canberra: A.N.U. Press, 1974), p. 83.

44. Goran Bratt-Venhalsan, Handout for Workshop I, Information Exchange: AIDS Conference of International Gay Association, Amsterdam, Jan. 20-22, 1984.

45. Sirois, "Epidemic Hysteria", *loc. cit.*, p. 25.

46. Figure 5: Samuel L. Maxwell, Jr., "Suicide by firearms", *N. Engl. J. Med.*, 1984; 310: 46-47. Figure 6: Compound graph derived from data contained in: M.A. Conant, *et al.*, "Changing Patterns of Sexually Transmitted Diseases over the Past 15 Years", in *AIDS: the Epidemic of Kaposi's Sarcoma and Opportunistic Infections*, ed. Alvin E. Friedman-Kien & Linda Laubenstein (New York: Masson, 1984), pp. 263-278.

47. *The Atlantic*, July 1984, cover.

48. *Time*, April 9, 1984, p. 61.

49. *The Observer*, October 30, 1983, p. 11.

50. George Will, *Newsweek*, November 7, 1983, p. 142.

51. William Fitch, *Christian Perspectives on Sex and Marriage* (Grand Rapids, Mich.: Eerdmans, 1971), p. 133.

52. Howard F. Stein, "Ethanol and its Discontents: Paradoxes of Inebriation and Sobriety in American Culture", *J. Psychoanal. Anthropol.*, 1982; 5: 355-377.

53. William R. Wedin, "No 'Cure' for Anonymous Sex", *New York Native*, April 9-22, 1984, pp. 21, 36. Also: "'Sexual Compulsion' — or, What's in a Name?: An Analysis of Anonymous Sexual Activity and Its Labelling", paper presented at the First International Lesbian and Gay Health Conference, New York, June 16, 1984.

54. Leo Srole with Anita Kassen Fischer, "The Midtown Manhattan Longitudinal Study vs. 'The Mental Paradise Lost' doctrine", *Arch Gen. Psychiatry*, 1980; 37: 209, 221. See also a corroborative study by the Wellesley College Center for Research on Women, showing that depression in women (ages 35-55) has declined dramatically: *U.S. News & World Report*, March 19, 1984, p. 47.

55. Paula Baker, "The Domestication of Politics: Women and American Political Society, 1780-1920", *Am. Hist. Rev.*, 1984; 89: 620-647, p. 638.

56. *Ladies' Home Journal*, January 1981, p. 32.

57. Natalie Gittelson, *Dominus: A Woman Looks at Men's Lives* (New York: Harcourt, Brace, Jovanovich, 1978).

58. *Ibid.*, p. 4.

59. *Ibid.*, p. 10.

60 *Ibid.*, p. 12.

61. *Ibid.*, p. 21.

62. *Ibid.*, p. 25.

63. Paul D. Meier, *Christian Child-Rearing and Personality Development* (Grand Rapids, Mich.: Baker Book House, 1977), p. 52.

64. See deMause, *Foundations*, pp. 188-192.

65. *Time*, April 9, 1984, p. 76.

66. *New York Native*, June 4-17, 1984, p. 15. The incident occurred on April 23, 1984.

67. *U.S. News & World Report*, October 31, 1977, p. 64.

68. Perry Deane Young, *God's Bullies: Native Reflections on Preachers and Politics* (New York: Holt, Rinehart & Winston, 1982), p. 92.

69. *Time*, August 2, 1982, cover.

70. *Time*, April 9, 1984, cover.

71. *Newsweek*, August 8, 1983, p. 30.

72. See: Casper G. Schmidt, "The Use of the Gallup Poll as a Psychohistorical Tool", *J. Psychohist.*, 1982; 10: 141-162.

73. Lloyd deMause, *Reagan's America* (New York: Creative Roots, 1984) pp. 51-67.

74. *Daily News*, July 20, 1984, p. 37.

75. *New York Native*, June 18-July 1, 1984, p. 27.

76. *Village Voice*, Voice Literary Supplement, June 1984, p. 16.

77. *Time*, June 4, 1984, p. 76.

78. Young, *op. cit.*, p. 270.

79. Dennis Altman, *The Homosexualization of America* (Boston: Beacon Press, 1982); John D'Emilio, *Sexual Politics, Sexual Communities: The Making of*

a Homosexual Minority in the United States, 1940-70 (Chicago: U. of Chicago Press, 1983).

80. *The Advocate*, August 11, 1976, p. 11.

81. *The Advocate*, May 7, 1975, p. 9.

82. Nathan Fain, "AIDS in the United States, Challenge and Response", European AIDS Conference, IGA, Amsterdam, January 20-22, 1984.

83. *The Advocate*, February 26, 1975, p. 17.

84. *The Advocate*, August 7, 1984, p. 25.

85. Howard F. Stein, "Judaism and the Group-Fantasy of Martyrdom: The Psychodynamic Paradox of Survival Through Persecution", *J. Psychohist.*, 1978; 6: 151-210.

86. *The Advocate*, July 28, 1976, p. 21.

87. *The Advocate*, March 23, 1977, p. 9.

88: *Ladies' Home Journal*, December 1980, p. 66.

89. *Ibid.*, p. 63.

90. Anita Bryant, *The Anita Bryant Story: The Survival of the Nation's Families and the Threat of Militant Homosexuality* (Old Tappan, N.J.: Fleming H. Revell Co., 1977), p. 53-54.

91. *Ibid.*, p. 55.

92. *Ibid.*, p. 55.

93. *Ibid.*, p. 59.

94. *Ibid.*, p. 91.

95. *Ibid.*, p. 89.

96. *Ibid.*, p. 111.

97. *Ibid.*, p. 116.

98. *Time*, June 20, 1977, p. 59.

99. *Time*, June 13, 1977, p. 20.

100. *Time*, June 20, 1977, p. 59.

101. *Ibid.*

102. *A note on countertransference:* I attempt to convey here an inkling of the tone of these events and the unspoken quiet horror that I imagine the recipients of these utterances must have felt. I felt myself pulled in three simultaneous directions as I was synthesising this section: identifications with all three groups of participants. At times it was hard for me to refrain from responding with revulsion and disgust at the cruelty of the New Right, just as I had to keep myself from sneering at the pathetic helplessness of the homosexuals, and just as I had to withhold myself from enjoying — with mainstream America — this moral slugfest as one would enjoy the gore in a Roman arena. I kept an even — though often unsteady — keel by remembering that all of these groups were desperately fighting for the integrity of their selves and their mental balance, and that they seemed only capable of doing so by viciously exploiting and abusing each other or themselves in their struggle for love.

103. Perry Deane Young, *op. cit.*, p. 308.

104. *Ibid.*, p. 221.

105. Fundraising letter for Christian Voice, n.d., signed by Robert G. Grant, cited in Alan Crawford, *Thunder on the Right: the "New right" and the Politics of Resentment* (New York: Pantheon, 1980), p. 146.

106. Young, *op.cit.*, p. 223.

107. *Ibid.*, p. 221.

108. *Ibid.*, p. 78.

109. *Ibid.*, p. 77.

110. Letha Scanzoni & Virginia Ramey Mollenkott, *Is the Homosexual My Neighbor?: Another Christian View* (New York: Harper & Row, 1978), p. 3.

111. Cited in Scanzoni, *op. cit.*, p. 7, from "Torture, Homosexuality, and the Cry for Hope", *The Other Side*, 1977; 13: 6.

112. Scanzoni, *op. cit.*, p. 31.

113. *Ibid.*, p. 32.

114. *Time*, June 13, 1977, p. 20.

CHAPTER II

Psychological and Toxicological Causes of "AIDS"[1]

John Lauritsen

Within a short time of our first meeting, I felt as though I had always known Casper Schmidt. For that matter, I can't remember exactly when or where we first met. It must have been in late 1987 or early 1988 — some time after I interviewed Peter Duesberg and was becoming known as an "AIDS dissident".

He was a brilliant man, knowledgeable in many different fields — charming and gracious, with a keen (and sometimes disconcerting) sense of humor — a loyal friend. I was very fond of him and miss him.

It would appear, at first glance, that my own approach to "AIDS" is very nearly the opposite of Casper Schmidt's — for my etiological model has consistently emphasized toxicology, while his emphasized psychology. In actuality, this was not the case, for we were in solid agreement on most matters, from the toxicities of AZT to the statistical prevarications of the CDC to the psychological characteristics of AIDS activists.

We never glossed over our differences. On some issues we agreed to disagree (which didn't preclude returning to them from time to time, if only for sport). On other issues we had a meeting of minds, and one or both of us modified our positions.

---

[1]Original for this book, though some material has previously been published.

This was certainly the case with my own multifactorial AIDS model, which acquired a psychological component under Casper Schmidt's tutelage. And in turn, Schmidt came to acknowledge the importance of toxicities in the syndrome, especially with regard to poppers (nitrite inhalants) and AZT.

In this essay I shall briefly present my own explanation of why some gay men, beginning in the late 70s and early 80s, became sick in ways that would be diagnosed as "AIDS".[2] This will involve looking closely at the gay subculture of the 70s, with the aim of identifying relevant health risks. I'll then compare my own latest model with Schmidt's as it developed.

Why are gay men becoming sick?

This is not the place to refute the HIV-AIDS hypothesis, which has been done elsewhere ... to the point of overkill and beyond.[3] Suffice it to say that HIV, as a biochemically inactive microbe, cannot be the cause of illness, "AIDS" or any other.

In criticism of the basic AIDS model, the question must be raised whether "AIDS" even exists as a coherent disease entity which can rationally be defined. People are undeniably sick, but are they sick with a new disease requiring its own name? It is my position that "AIDS" exists only as a construct, which spuriously links 29 (at last count) old and extremely heterogeneous "AIDS-

---

[2]My most comprehensive model is "The Risk-AIDS Hypothesis", one of the key chapters of my book, *The AIDS War*. In addition to discussing the causes of AIDS-illnesses in gay men (the basis of much of the present essay), this chapter deals at length with the other "risk groups": intravenous drug users, hemophiliacs, transfusion cases, and inhabitants of Africa.

[3]See Appendix A.

indicator diseases" together with a presumption of HIV infection. (I put "AIDS" in quotation marks to emphasize that its sole reality is that of a construct.) In almost all cases, the presumed HIV infection is nothing more than a positive reading on one or both of the unvalidated and unreliable "HIV-antibody" tests.[4]

After rejecting the hypothesis that HIV is pathogenic, as well as the hypothesis that "AIDS" exists as a coherent disease entity, one is left with the risk groups and their illnesses. I shall argue that the health risks affecting a certain subset of gay men are extremely serious, readily apparent once one is willing to look at them, and entirely sufficient to cause illnesses that earn an "AIDS" diagnosis.

Although gay men currently comprise 58% of the cumulative "AIDS" cases in the U.S., as a whole they are not at risk for developing "AIDS".[5] All across America are tens of millions of males who have had sex with each other, and who remain healthy.

There is nothing wrong with all-male sex, though like anything else it should be conducted in accordance with common sense and rational ethical standards. Male love is inherently good — for body and mind. In ancient Greece, the birthplace of Western Civilization, it was considered the highest form of love, practised by the leading citizens and by the gods themselves.

---

[4]See Eleopulos-Papadopulos *et al.*, Appendix A.

[5]By the end of 1995, "AIDS" diagnoses had been given to over half a million (506,538) American adults and adolescents, of whom 58% were gay men. The 58% can be broken down into those who had used IV drugs (7%) and those who had not used IV drugs (51%). *CDC AIDS Surveillance Report — Year-end 1995 Edition,* Vol. 7, No. 2.

The ultimate source of the gay health crisis is the theological prohibition of sex between males — a taboo formulated 2500 years ago by the Levites, the priestly class of the tribe of Judah, as part of their *Holiness Code* (which also includes hundreds of taboos against foods, forms of clothing, divers sexual acts, and all kinds of other things).[6] The Levitical taboo was evaluated by the philosopher Bertrand Russell in the following terms:

> Every person who has taken the trouble to study the subject knows that this law [against male-male sex] is the effect of a barbarous and ignorant superstition in favour of which no rational argument of any sort or kind can be advanced.[7]

This taboo on all-male sex — not a whit more rational than the taboo on eating pork — was carried forward by Christians and Jews alike to become an unquestioned part of the culture we live in. Over the centuries it has caused suffering and death for males who were lovers of their own kind, from the persecutions under the early Christian emperors to the Inquisitions of the middle ages to the AIDS holocaust of the present.

It is only a very small, particular subset of gay men who are getting sick, and they are getting sick for reasons that are all too

---

[6]*Leviticus* 020:013 King James Version: "If a man also lie with mankind, as he lieth with a woman, both of them have committed an abomination: they shall surely be put to death; their blood shall be upon them."

[7]World League for Sexual Reform, *Proceedings of 1929 London Congress*. Cited in: John Lauritsen and David Thorstad, *The Early Homosexual Rights Movement (1864-1935)*, New York 1974; Second, revised edition, Ojai, California 1995.

obvious once the right questions are asked. Before going into greater detail, let me simply list the major health risks impinging on those gay men who are getting sick:

- "Recreational" drugs
- Medical drugs (especially including the nucleoside analogue drugs: AZT, ddI, ddC, d4T, d3T, *etc.*)
- Repeated infections with sexually transmitted diseases, treated with antibiotics
- Psychological factors.

On the surface it would seem that these particular health risks do not affect only gay men. However, a closer examination shows that within each of these risk categories there are elements peculiar to a subset of gay men, in terms of both intensity and specificity.

The following profile[8] fits most, if not necessarily all, gay men who have developed "AIDS": In the decade preceding their diagnosis they contracted venereal diseases many times, treated with ever stronger doses of antibiotics; they took antibiotics prophylactically, to avoid getting VD again; they drank too much; they used "recreational" drugs; they smoked heavily; they

---

[8]I have developed this profile from my own interviews with many dozens of gay men with "AIDS"; from direct observation; from survey research (however inadequate); from discussions with leaders in the People With AIDS Coalition and its predecessor, Gay Men With AIDS, Positively Healthy, HEAL, and Continuum; and from the reminiscences of those who observed "the scene".

experienced terror, owing to a war waged against gay men by religious bigots; they experienced loneliness, alienation, and depression; they experienced shame and self-hatred, which, in a vicious circle, they acted out in ways that degraded themselves — and, as the epidemic developed, they experienced grief: they were in perpetual mourning, their hearts broken by the loss of their closest friends.

Following the Stonewall Rebellion of 1969, and the Gay Liberation Movement, a gay sex industry mushroomed, bringing with it a lifestyle which many gay men adopted as their own: the "Gay Clone" lifestyle. Suddenly, in every area of life, men who defined themselves as "gay" differentiated themselves from the "straights". There were gay baths, sex clubs, restaurants, drugs, clothes, music, grooming styles, facial expressions, gestures, language, publications, pornography, and so on.

As a precursor to the mass sacrificial ritual described so vividly by Casper Schmidt, many gay men who "came out" in the 70s succumbed to an intense herd mentality. They became, as the word "clone" implies, extreme conformists — devotees of a religion whose dogmas and observances were still being formed.[9] To be sure, there were still gay individualists and lone wolves, but their activities and aspirations were inundated in the wave of commercialized gregariousness that followed the Stonewall Rebellion.[10]

---

[9]Observers in London have told me that, for the first few years of the AIDS epidemic, virtually all of the victims were "Scene Queans" (that is, gay men whose lives revolved around the gay discos and other aspects of the "gay scene").

[10]Changes wrought by gay liberation are described in Ian Young's book, *The Stonewall Experiment: A Gay Psychohistory*, London and New York 1995.

One might have thought that gay liberation would usher in a new era of sexual freedom and happiness, but this did not happen. Sexuality itself was reduced to fleeting encounters in baths or pitch-dark back rooms. In the latter environment, sexual partners were not spoken to, or even seen, let alone confronted as complete human beings — or indeed, as complete human bodies. Some gay men never learned to make love, but instead came to define their sexual identity in terms of a bizarre and fragmentary repertoire of *acts*. They became adepts at performing skin piercing, "tit jobs", "rimming", enemas, "golden showers", "fist fucking", "scat", and other acts they had learned from hard-core porn or S&M/leather publications.[11] Their sexuality, which should have been an expression of strength and joy, was expressed in ways that were morbid and unfulfilling.

The commercial gay clone subculture was in many ways unhealthful and dehumanizing.[12] With the gay bar as the primary meeting place, many men became alcoholics. Excessively

---

[11]"Fist fucking" consists of inserting a hand into someone's rectum. The practice is extremely dangerous, and a number of people die from it every year, though the cause of death is almost always covered up. In one of the early studies of gay men with "AIDS", a third of the sample admitted to having been fist fucked. Those who get fist fucked are heavily reliant upon drugs — especially poppers, which relax the sphincter muscle and deaden the sense of pain.

[12]At some level of consciousness the interior decorators of the gay establishments apprehended the morbidity of these places. Eric Bernard, an interior decorator who died of "AIDS", pioneered the concept of the all-black interior. The idea took hold in the gay community, and by the late 70s (a few years before the first cases of "AIDS" began to appear) an all-black interior was a strong indicator of a gay establishment, whether bar, bathhouse, porn theatre, sex shop, club, or discotheque. Walls, ceilings, and everything else would be black, the color of death.

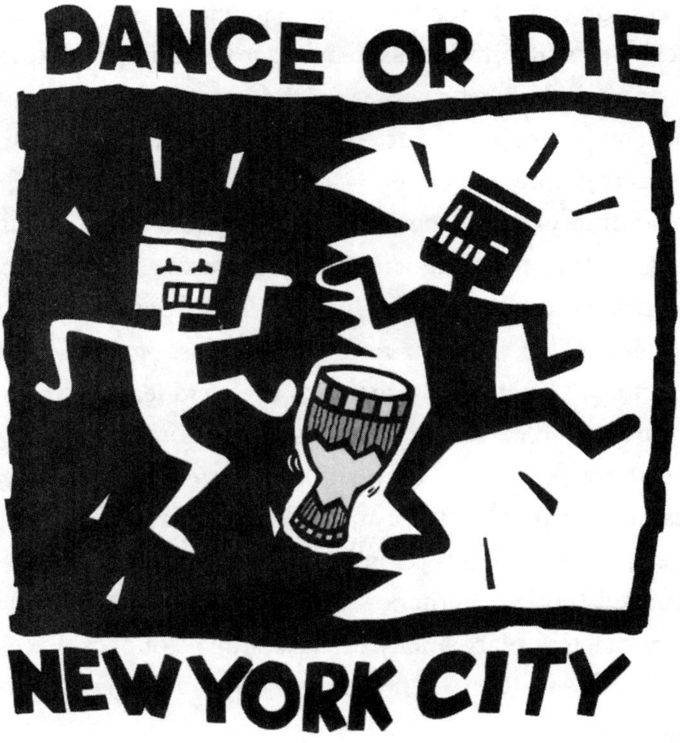

Disco was, like the medieval *Totentanz* or *Danse Macabre,* a dance led by Death. This T-shirt design is either by or in the style of Keith Haring, who died of "AIDS"/AZT poisoning in 1990. It captures the hellishly driven character of the gay disco ritual. The utter joylessness of the experience is conveyed by the grimaces of the deaths-head dancers, who can find no rest from the inexorable, computer-generated beat.

An observer of the scene, whose mind was not befuddled by drugs, would have perceived that the energy displayed by a few dancers was not accompanied by any sign of genuine and spontaneous pleasure. He'd have seen that most of the men present were in a state of drug-induced stupor. And he'd have noticed the lack of human interaction — the obligatory separation of the dancers, as though they were forbidden to touch each other.

loud sound systems prevented socializing through the oldest of barroom pastimes, *conversation.* At gay discos, regular and prolonged exposure to pain-threshold noise posed serious health hazards (stress, immunosuppression, and premature deafness). Promiscuity led to frequent infection and re-infection with a wide spectrum of venereal diseases, including syphilis, gonorrhea, amoebiasis, chlamydia, hepatitis, CMV, etc. Not only were frequent treatments with antibiotics necessary, but some men began taking them prophylactically: they would swallow a handful before going to the baths. Inadequate sleep, malnutrition, and feelings of alienation, loneliness, and low self-esteem were concomitants of the lifestyle.

The bars and other gay establishments that existed prior to Stonewall were not ideal. They were often dark, dirty, and subject to police raids. But at least they afforded gay men a place to meet each other and socialize. And the best of them had warmth. Juke boxes offered a variety of music, including such favorites as Edith Piaf, Bobby Short, Chris Conner, Billy Holliday, Frank Sinatra — and in time, rock & roll, twist, *etc.* The guys cruised each other, and went home together, but they also talked to each other, sometimes for hours. In contrast, from the mid-70s onwards the bars and discos played *only* disco — a soulless and mechanical noise — and this at high volume. In purely practical terms it is difficult to introduce one's self to someone, or converse with him, if it's necessary to shout in his ear just to be heard over the din of the disco.

Some establishments in New York City and San Francisco provided a Theater of Depravity, which encouraged the patrons to abuse each other psychologically and physically. There were sex clubs featuring rooms in which demented beings in bath tubs waited for others to come along and use them as toilets. Some places featured slings, in which the occupants became communal semen receptacles. One "Black Party" at a popular disco club provided, for entertainment, the spectacle of a young man mutilating himself and of a pig being slaughtered. This syndrome of recreational abuse was satirized by Hot Peaches in one of their songs from the mid-70s, which, as my memory serves me, had such lines as: "Use me, abuse me ... I want to be sleazy!".

I have described these things, neither to condemn nor to titillate, but to make a point, which is important: *The commercial gay milieu was extremely unhealthy psychologically* — aside from and in addition to the specific health risks (drugs and disease) that were teeming within it.

Inextricably bound up with the physical components of addiction are the psychological. Foremost is *denial:* the lies an addict tells himself and others in order to conceal, rationalize, and ultimately sustain his addiction. Denial of the role of VD and drugs in making gay men sick has insidiously undermined efforts to formulate rational treatment and prevention guidelines.

In the past decade I have spoken before hundreds of people with "AIDS" diagnoses (PWAs for short). Always I have asked if there were any to whom my risk-profile did not apply. The overwhelming audience response has been that the profile was right on target. I have encountered only a handful of exceptions. One man said he had not used drugs (other than moderate amounts of poppers and marijuana); it turned out he didn't have "AIDS", but was merely HIV-positive. The others were not speaking about themselves — to whom the profile *did* apply — but about friends or acquaintances they imagined were "not like that". In every case, further questioning brought out that they knew almost nothing about the other person's use of drugs, sexual history, or psychological state.

Possibly no one personally knew more PWAs than Michael Callen, one of the founders of the People With AIDS Coalition. At the time of his death, on 27 December 1993, Callen had survived over eleven years with a diagnosis of "AIDS". His good-natured skepticism enabled him to penetrate smokescreens of denial on the part of other PWAs:

> I have gone to a great deal of trouble to find these people who claim to have had only one or two "unlucky" sexual contacts. I found ten of them in all, and each one ended up telling me they had been lying. I've known several people who were saying, in public, "I only had one or two contacts". "I only had one lover and we were monogamous", but then in the support group setting, they would regale us with tales of bathhouses and promiscuity and lovers on the side and drug use.[13]

When I spoke to Michael Callen not quite a year before his death, I asked him if he had ever encountered a gay male PWA who did not fit the profile of venereal diseases, antibiotics, drugs, and stress. His answer was: "No. Not in eleven years."[14]

Now, let's take a closer look at drug abuse among gay men, beginning with the premier gay drug, "poppers". Almost all gay men, but few other people, know what poppers are: little bottles containing a liquid mixture of isobutyl nitrite and other chemicals. When inhaled just before orgasm, poppers seem to enhance

---

[13]Celia Farber, interview with Michael Callen, "AIDS: Words from the Front", *SPIN*, June 1988.

[14]Telephone conversation, 21 January 1993.

and prolong the sensation. Poppers facilitate anal intercourse by relaxing the muscles in the rectum and deadening the sense of pain.

The original poppers were little glass ampules enclosed in mesh, which were "popped" under the nose and inhaled. Manufactured by Burroughs-Wellcome, of AZT notoriety, they contained pharmaceutical amyl nitrite, and were intended for emergency relief of angina pectoris (heart pain). Amyl nitrite was a controlled substance until 1960, when the prescription requirement was eliminated by the Food and Drug Administration (FDA). From 1961 to 1969, a few gay men, primarily those into S&M (sadomasochism), began using amyl nitrite as a "recreational" drug. The prescription requirement was reinstated by the FDA in 1969.

In 1970, a new industry stepped into the breach, marketing brands of butyl and isobutyl nitrite. One of the most brilliant advertising campaigns of all time commenced. Within only a few years hundreds of thousands of men were persuaded that poppers were an integral part of their own "gay identity". The ads conveyed the message that nothing could be butcher or sexier than to inhale noxious chemical fumes. Bulging muscles were linked to a drug that is indisputably hazardous to the health.

At its peak, the poppers industry was the biggest money-maker in the gay business world, grossing upwards of $50 million per year. Gay publications were delighted with the revenues they received from running full-page, four-color ads for the various brands of poppers. In a 1983 letter to the *Advocate*, poppers manufacturer Joseph F. Miller, President of Great Lakes Products, Inc., boasted he was the "largest advertiser in the Gay press".

By 1974 the poppers craze was in full swing, and by 1977 poppers were in every corner of gay life. At gay discotheques men could be seen shuffling around in a daze, holding popper bottles under the nose. At gay gathering places — bars, baths, leather clubs — the miasma of volatile nitrites was taken for granted. Some gay men became so addicted to poppers that they were never without their little bottle, from which they snorted nitrite fumes around the clock.

For gay men who came out in the 70s, poppers appeared to be as much a part of the gay clone lifestyle as mustaches or flannel shirts. The brilliant red and yellow label of one brand, Rush®, was so distinctive that a successful gay political candidate in San Francisco used the color scheme on his campaign posters. Accessories were marketed: for leather queans, there were little metal inhalers on leather thongs. One magazine had a comic strip entitled "Poppers"; its hero, Billy, was a child-like but sexy blond, whose two main loves in life were sex and poppers.

In 1981 Hank Wilson in San Francisco noticed that many of his popper-using friends were developing swollen lymph nodes. After reading medical literature on the nitrite inhalants, which was extensive even then, he founded the Committee to Monitor the Cumulative Effects of Poppers. I began collaborating with Wilson in 1983, and in 1986 we published a book together.[15]

Poppers are hazardous to the health in many different ways: They damage the immune system. They cause anemia (both Heinz body hemolytic anemia and methemoglobinemia). They damage the lungs. Poppers are strongly mutagenic (that is, they cause cellular mutations), and they have the potential to cause cancer by producing deadly N-nitroso compounds. Poppers can cause serious skin burns and death or brain damage from

---

[15]John Lauritsen and Hank Wilson, *Death Rush: Poppers & AIDS*, New York 1986.

cardiovascular collapse or stroke.[16] Poppers have been used successfully to commit suicide (by drinking) and murder. (The victim was gagged with a sock soaked with poppers.)

There are strong epidemiological links between the use of poppers and the development of AIDS, especially Kaposi's sarcoma (KS).[17] In AIDS cases, KS is found almost entirely among gay men who used poppers, not among members of other "risk groups". A six-fold decrease in the incidence of KS over the past five years parallels a sharp decline in the use of poppers.[18]

Many drugs other than poppers were a familiar part of the gay scene. Studies conducted by the CDC in 1981 and 1982 showed extremely heavy use of non-injected drugs among gay men with "AIDS", with 17% of the sample having used intravenous drugs as well.[19] A squeamishness regarding the use of needles may be one difference between fast-lane gay men and their straight counterparts. W.J. Wallace, manager of The Mineshaft, stated in 1984: "I really don't know anybody who's had AIDS who hasn't

---

[16]See Appendix B.

[17]A blood vessel abnormality. It is now known that Kaposi's sarcoma, despite its name, is *not* a cancer.

[18]The argument that the volatile nitrites cause KS among gay men is powerful from the standpoint of epidemiology (the strong correlation between nitrite inhalant usage and KS) and also from the standpoint of biochemistry: poppers are a potent mutagen and affect the blood vessels. It is suggestive, to say the least, that many gay men who used poppers developed KS of the upper lips, nose, and lungs — the route of poppers inhalation.

[19]The studies are discussed in Chapter I: "CDC's Tables Obscure AIDS-Drug Connection", in *The AIDS War.*

used drugs." He later expanded on this statement in a letter to the *New York Native:*

> At the time of that interview, poppers was not included as one of the drugs we were discussing. We were talking about the use of downers and uppers, ethel chloride, THC, MDA, black beauties, LSD, microdots, and other homemade concoctions and black market (often outdated) pharmaceutical items, which are far more common to the gay lifestyle than intravenous drugs. Many gay men are appalled at the thought of sticking a needle in their arms, but think nothing of popping the pill that is the "in" high. Why more attention in research and public warnings has not been paid to these "little goodies", I do not know. Example: Why does the Safe Sex Poster we are requested to hang under glass in our club fail to warn people against drug usage? Strange, isn't it?
>
> — W.J. Wallace, Manager, The Mineshaft[20]

In his pre-AIDS novel, *Faggots*, Larry Kramer provides a list of the favorite drugs of the Fire Island set:

> MDA, MDM, THC, PCP, STP, DMT, LDK, WDW, Coke, Window Pane, Blotter, Orange Sunshine, Sweet Pea, Sky Blue, Christmas Tree, Mescalin, Dust, Benzedrine, Dexedrine, Dexamyl, Desoxyn, Strychnine, Ionamin, Ritalin, Desbutal, Opitol, Glue, Ethyl Chloride, Nitrous Oxide, Crystal Methedrine, Clogidal, Nesperan, Tytch, Nestex, Black Beauty, Certyn, Preludin with B-12, Zayl ... Quaalude, Tuinal, Nembutal,

---

[20]W.J. Wallace, "The Mineshaft and Poppers", letter to the *New York Native*, 26 August - 1 September 1985.

> Seconal, Amytal, Phenobarb, Elavil, Valium, Librium, Darvon, Mandrax, Desnobarb, Opium, Stidyl, Halidax, Calcifyn, Optimil, Drayl ... Magic ... grasses: Mexican, Jamaican, Colombian, Thai, Pakistani, Lower Urdu ... Moroccan Hash, Red Lebanese, Black Afghani, Hawaiian, Kentucky Bluegrass, Bridgeport Blunder, Mantanuska Thunderfuck, Wildbush, Black African, American First. [p. 236]

Apparently Kramer didn't think poppers even counted as drugs, as they are conspicuously absent from his list.

An article on gay drug abuse by George De Stefano provides a vignette of a disco devotee:

> Fred is highly agitated, seemingly on the verge of tears. Stoned when he arrived at the club several hours earlier, he has misplaced a stash of several hundred dollars worth of "disco drugs" — MDA, Ecstasy, speed, coke. Did he lose it in the taxi on the way to The Saint? Did it fall out when he reached into his pocket for the cab fare? He's gone through his coat and gym bag, which he retrieved from his locker, and he has thoroughly searched the locker room. "I can't believe I lost my drugs", Fred wails, "This is the second time this month!" The only intoxicant he's got left is the ethyl chloride-soaked rag he's been sucking on while dancing. After uttering more lamentations over his loss, he wads the rag into his mouth and heads back to the dance floor. Fred is a successful psychiatrist with a predominantly gay practice. He has, however, lost a shockingly high number of clients to AIDS.[21]

---

[21] George De Stefano, "Gay Drug Abuse: Owning Up to a Serious Problem", *The Advocate,* 24 June 1986.

Tribal Rites, a collection of reminiscences of the gay disco scene in San Francisco, makes it apparent that drugs were every bit as important there as in New York.[22] One difference between the two cities is that sexual activity took place in the New York dance clubs, but not those in San Francisco. People went to the latter only to dance — and do drugs. Though some of the voices in *Tribal Rites* recall their disco experiences as the happiest of their life, they are saddened that by 1987 many of the important disco people — producers, performers, and DJs — had already died of "AIDS". To the disco aficionados, a night at the Trocadero or Dreamland was more than a form of entertainment; it was, in their words, a "religious experience". They still do not realize that their "church" was a death cult.

Group activity was the essence of the gay disco ritual. If something was done, everybody did it. At a disco like The Saint, several thousand gay men would be on the same drug at the same time. An hour or so later, word would get around that it was "Special K time", and everybody would go on that. And still other drugs would be taken in their appointed time.

This is the kind of drug abuse that took place among fast-lane gay men in the 70s and 80s, just before the appearance of "AIDS". The existing medical literature is hopelessly inadequate to evaluate the consequences of such prodigious chemical intake. No one (except perhaps for a few underground chemists) even knows what many of the drugs were. (A special acid was prepared only once for the opening of The Saint.) There is precious little literature on the long-term consequences of any of the "gay drugs". And there would be no way that the drug-

---

[22]David Diebold, *Tribal Rites: A Forum on the San Francisco Dance Music Phenomenon 1977-1987*, San Francisco 1987.

interaction effects of the drugs could be studied, given the custom of taking a half dozen different drugs in the course of an evening. Is it likely that any researcher will conduct a study to evaluate the long-term toxicities of poppers, MDA, quaaludes, LSD, alcohol, cocaine and Special K in combination? The only thing of which we can be sure is that this kind of drug abuse is very bad for the health.

Now let's move on to examine venereal diseases and antibiotics as risk factors. Early studies of gay men with "AIDS" indicated that the patients, on the average, had been extremely promiscuous.[23] A typical medical history would include dozens of cases of VD in the decade before the "AIDS" diagnosis. Each case of VD would be treated with stronger and stronger doses of antibiotics. Some doctors gave their gay patients open prescriptions for antibiotics, advising them to swallow a few before going to the baths. One popular bath house in New York (now closed) sold black market tetracycline on the second floor, along with all kinds of street drugs.

In the early days of the epidemic, one etiological hypothesis was "immunological overload". The idea was that under repeated and multiple cases of infectious disease — hepatitis, cytomegalovirus, herpes simplex, gonorrhea, syphilis, chlamydia, *etc.* — the immune system was battered down until it collapsed irreversibly. There is no doubt an element of truth in the hypothesis. Diseases

[23]See, for example, Harold Jafee *et al.*, "National Case-Control Study of Kaposi's Sarcoma and Pneumocystis carinii Pneumonia in Homosexual Men: Part 1, Epidemiologic Results", *Annals of Internal Medicine,* August 1983. A typical government study, this is far below the standards of professional survey research; it contains some useful information, but ridiculous conclusions. I have critiqued it briefly in Chapter XIV: "Incompetence in AIDS Epidemiology" in *Poison By Prescription: The AZT Story.*

take their toll on the body, and no rational person would allow himself to contract VD all the time. However, there is a blind spot, especially among physicians, regarding the role of medical treatments in making people sick.

Antibiotics first came into clinical use in the 1940s, which means that human beings and all other animal species have experienced them for no more than half a century, out of millions of years of evolution. By the time it is possible fully to evaluate the long-term consequences of antibiotics, it may be too late. Almost every physician I have spoken to has put forward the Pollyanna platitude that *antibiotics merely assist the body in fighting infection*. In fact, some antibiotics, like Chloromycetin, can have very serious side effects.[24]

Experimental pathologist Marc Lappé makes the case[25] that the misuse of antibiotics poses a grave threat to all of us:

> By making our own bodies the battle grounds for chemical control of bacteria, we disrupt the natural ecological balance of the microorganisms that maintain the homeostasis of our internal and external surfaces.... Overuse of antibiotics like penicillin may have participated in creating the soil for

---

[24]For background on dangerous antibiotics and other drugs, read Morton Mintz, *By Prescription Only (A report on the United States Food and Drug Administration, the American Medical Association, pharmaceutical manufacturers, and others in connection with the irrational and massive use of prescription drugs that may be worthless, injurious, or even lethal)*, Boston, 1967; and James S. Turner, *The Chemical Feast: The Ralph Nader Study Group Report on Food Protection and the Food and Drug Administration*, New York, 1970.

[25]Marc Lappé, *When Antibiotics Fail: Restoring the Ecology of the Body*, Berkeley 1986.

epidemics of antibiotic-resistant bacteria, and perhaps even AIDS.

If antibiotics represent a health threat to ordinary people, then they must represent an immeasurably greater threat to the health of those gay men who took massive doses of them for years. One PWA told me that, from the time he was prescribed tetracycline for acne at the age of 14, there had never been a day in his life when he was not on antibiotics.

Yeast or fungal infections are an expected consequence of treatment with broad-spectrum antibiotics like tetracycline, which destroy the friendly bacteria that normally keep such funguses as *Candida albicans* in check. Since "candidiasis of bronchi, trachea, or lungs" and "candidiasis of esophagus" are two of the "AIDS-indicator diseases", and since antibiotics cause candidiasis, it logically follows that antibiotics can cause "AIDS" (provided, of course, that HIV be either detected *or presumed*). In addition to candidiasis, other fungal infections that qualify as AIDS-indicator diseases include cryptococcosis, coccidioidomycosis, and histoplasmosis. Some researchers also consider pneumocystis carinii pneumonia and toxoplasmosis to be fungal diseases.

Systemic infection with *Candida albicans* can cause a "yeast syndrome", which weakens the health in general and the immune system in particular. One authority on candidiasis had this to say in 1982:

> *Candida albicans* seems to be at least one agent capable of at least a depressing, and perhaps a destructive effect on the immune system. Until the cause of the AIDS problem is un-

covered, any approach would seem to be worth considering in a situation of such urgency.[26]

In addition to antibiotics, many gay men in the 70s and 80s were treated for amebiasis with toxic anti-parasite drugs such as Flagyl, a carcinogen, and diiodohydroxyquin (brand name Diodoquin), which is closely related to a drug that causes nerve damage resulting in paralysis, blindness, and death.[27]

Psychological factors also play a role in making gay men sick, as Casper Schmidt and Ian Young have eloquently argued. A sacrificial ritual was indeed taking place — and the sites for the ritual were such places as The Saint, The Mineshaft, The Toilet, Trocadero, Flamingo — everywhere that gay men took poison communion or flagellated themselves physically and psychologically.

The bottom line is that there were abundant health risks in the lives of those gay men who developed "AIDS", and it would have been amazing if any of them had remained healthy.

Casper Schmidt's model revisited

"The Group-Fantasy Origins of AIDS" was the first major critique of the orthodox AIDS paradigm. Considering that the essay was written in 1984, before the "AIDS Virus" had been baptized as the "Human Immunodeficiency Virus" (HIV), it

---

[26]C. Orian Truss, quoted in William G. Crook's *The Yeast Connection: A Medical Breakthrough,* New York 1986 (updated and revised edition).

[27]Discussed in Excursus 6: "The SMON Story" in *The AIDS War* and also in Peter Duesberg's *Inventing the AIDS Virus* (see Appendix A).

stands up remarkably well. Every time I re-read it I am impressed by the grand depiction of historical circumstances, the wealth of anthropological and psychological analogies, the keen insights, and the unique combination of irony and compassion.

Future historians will have to grapple with the question of how the U.S. Public Health Service and the medical establishments of the entire world could have gone so disastrously wrong. How could people of the late 20th century ever have believed anything so manifestly preposterous as the now-prevailing AIDS myths? I believe that they will find answers to at least the psychosocial aspects of these questions in Casper Schmidt's early essay.

The AIDS phenomenon changed very rapidly and dramatically after 1984. Initially Schmidt and I disagreed on whether "AIDS" really existed as a disease entity, or whether (as I argued) it was merely a construct. Our disagreement on this issue shrank as the Centers for Disease Control (CDC) expanded its surveillance definition of "AIDS" again and again. In 1984 most "AIDS" diagnoses were based on a diagnosis of Kaposi's sarcoma (an affliction of the blood vessels) or pneumocystis carinii pneumonia (a lung disease caused by the overgrowth of a ubiquitous microbe) along with a presumption of "immune deficiency" and a presumption of retroviral infection. When the CDC expanded the list of "AIDS-indicator diseases" in 1987, it caused an immediate boost of new AIDS cases by approximately one-third. Using the pre-1987 definition, the incidence of new "AIDS" cases peaked in 1988, but with the net cast ever wider, incidence continued to rise ... at least for a few years. In early 1992 still more "AIDS-indicator diseases" were added to the list, bringing the total to 29, and reducing the AIDS-construct to utter absurdity. In 1982 someone who earned an "AIDS" diagnosis was very close to death; after 1992 someone could acquire an "AIDS" diagnosis without even being sick.[28]

I can still remember Schmidt's contempt for the CDC's tactics in adding cervical cancer to the list in 1992. As might be expected, the revision caused an immediate rise in "AIDS" diagnoses among women, enabling the CDC to issue press releases proclaiming that *AIDS was spreading fastest among heterosexual women.*

Another change in the AIDS phenomenon since 1984 has been the phenomenal growth of a multi-billion dollar AIDS industry, which comprises pharmaceutical companies, condom manufacturers, the latex industry, AIDS organizations of every imaginable description, viatical settlement companies (which purchase the life insurance policies of terminally sick people), biotechnology, retrovirology, hospitals, counsellors, social workers, and much more. Once tens of billions of dollars had been invested in the HIV-Causes-AIDS hypothesis, it was no longer something that could lightly be discarded, no matter how flimsy it was and is when judged by standards of logic and evidence.

Still another change in the AIDS phenomenon concerns the emergence of iatrogenic "AIDS" — that is, "AIDS" caused by the administration of AZT and other nucleoside analogue drugs to people who are HIV-antibody positive but objectively healthy. Since AZT can directly cause several of the "AIDS-indicator diseases", and can probably contribute indirectly to most of the

---

[28]A CD-4 cell count of less than 200 per milliliter is one of the official "AIDS-indicator diseases", although there is no reliable statistical evidence that such a count is not compatible with perfectly good health.

others, it logically follows that AZT can cause "AIDS".[29] Indeed, the package insert for AZT — written by the manufacturer to present the drug as favorably as possible — states that the symptoms of AIDS and the toxicities of AZT are similar.

Schmidt was horrified by the mass administration of AZT (a failed cancer chemotherapy drug, designed to kill growing cells through the termination of DNA synthesis), and he forcefully spoke out against it on many occasions. One evening in New York City, as he and I were leaving a meeting of the Act Up Treatment & Data Committee, he told me that he finally understood the psychology of these "AIDS activists". "They *know* that AZT is poison", he said, "they know that it's poison, and they want it *because* it's poison!"

The psychological factors making gay men sick increased greatly since 1984, as discussed in the other essays in this book. Gay men were programmed by the AIDS Establishment to become sick; they were provided with a schedule, told not only that they *ought* to become sick, but exactly *how* and *when* to become sick.

Over the centuries gay men have been outcasts in societies governed by Judeo-Christian morality. The companionship of their own kind made it easier to bear this onus. Against a hostile world they found solace in each other's arms. AIDS propaganda changed this: it killed love. The deepest relationship in life became fraught with fear and suspicion, and the fellowship of gay men increasingly became one of mutual support for victimhood.

---

[29] "AIDS" is defined by the formula: AIDS-Indicator Disease + HIV = AIDS. When an "asymptomatic" HIV-positive person begins AZT therapy, he has already met the second condition of the formula. Only an "AIDS-indicator disease" is then needed for him to achieve an official "AIDS" diagnosis.

It would be fallacious to counterpose psychological and toxicological explanations for why gay men are becoming sick; the two go together. It is impossible to understand substance abuse without taking into account the concomitant social and psychological issues, regardless of how toxic and addictive the substance in question may be. At the same time, extreme psychological states can cause chemical changes in the body, as discussed by Casper Schmidt in his interview with Ian Young, and can cause behavioral changes with health implications.

Mind and Body form a unity, which cannot be disregarded in understanding the causes of "AIDS" and other illnesses. In 1993 I wrote a program for recovery from "AIDS", based on my own analysis of the health risks I have described above, as well as the practical examples of those who are returning to health after receiving "AIDS" diagnoses.[30] In a nutshell, I said that a PWA should ruthlessly identify all health risks in his life and then take appropriate action. Body and mind should be detoxified, the body should be allowed to heal itself, the PWA should expect a return to health, and so on. I have become less optimistic since then, as the realization has sunk in that some gay men have long ago said *no* to life, an orientation not easily reversed.

Casper Schmidt's depiction of gay men as "willing sacrificial victims" is one I have observed in person more than once, an uncanny experience. An HIV-positive man in his thirties will be speaking to me. He seems to grasp my arguments, and then suddenly a meek and stubborn fatalism takes over — he dons the Mantle of AIDS — his aura becomes fey, bleak and withdrawn. Communication is over, and anger will flare up at any attempt

---

[30]Chapter XX: "Recovery From AIDS" in *The AIDS War.*

to awaken him from his trance. He will not be dissuaded from proceeding with his cohort to the sacrificial altar — which in practical terms means taking the latest drug "cocktail" being touted by the AIDS Establishment.

Alcoholics Anonymous literature describes alcoholism as "a three-fold disease: mental, physical, and spiritual". The same applies to many PWAs, who are suffering as much from soul-sickness as from immune deficiency. For them, recovery may very well require a total transformation of attitudes and philosophy: a miracle. Medical people don't like to hear talk like this, but it is true. All the medical technology in the world cannot help someone who has lost the desire to live. Nor is there any pharmaceutical quick fix for a person whose life is in shambles and whose behavior is self-destructive.

The AIDS organizations, including such pseudo-radical groups as Act Up, are always demanding a "cure" for AIDS. By "cure" they mean a new, high-tech drug that will attack HIV. This is understandable, but misguided.

What people living with an "HIV-positive" or an "AIDS" diagnosis need, is not a new drug, but a counsellor with a clear mind and a warm heart. They need someone who will treat them as a whole person, not as a patient labelled with particular diagnoses. They need a friend, who will help them put their lives in order, and who will guide them back to the path of good health.

CHAPTER III

Lessons From Hiroshima[1]

George N. Hazlehurst

In 1955, during a two-year stint as internist with the Atomic Bomb Casualty Commission in Hiroshima studying the *late effects*[2] of radiation on the citizens exposed to the atomic bomb ten years previously, I made what I considered to be an important discovery. I had been told before I went to Japan that the death rate was twice as great in the exposed population as in the control (unexposed) population, and no one knew why. In-depth conversations with some of the survivors, however, revealed the strong belief that each one's life would be shortened as the result of exposure to the bomb. This was also the belief of neighbors who were not exposed, but who moved to Hiroshima later on, and in many cases stigmatized the survivors as doomed and subjected them to ostracism in regard to association or intermarriage. These fears were also supported by doctors in the community who touted A-bomb disease as death cause for anyone exposed who died of *any cause*. Also, public exhibits sponsored by the Commission exaggerated in citizens' minds possible diseases

[1]This essay has circulated in manuscript form, but is previously unpublished.

[2]Not to be confused with *early effects* of radiation injury, or "radiation sickness", which occurs within one to three weeks after exposure, and is self-limited either by death from massive exposure or, for survivors, an illness lasting from a few weeks to several months, with eventual full recovery.

caused by atomic bomb exposure, e.g., a small but statistically significant increase in leukemia, unduly adding to the people's anxiety. Belief in early death was seen to be widespread in the population, and my contention was that such a strongly held belief could actually bring about early death, no matter the final real cause.

Belief in early death as *cause* of early death could not be accepted by the medical staff then in 1955, nor is the idea generally acceptable by scientific types now nearly 40 years later, although many doctors at present embrace the idea that one's attitude can influence one's health in many ways, and are saying so in a number of recent books. My request to continue the work interviewing the survivors in depth (with an excellent interpreter) to further explore feelings and attitudes was denied, and so the work had to be halted in its beginnings. Efforts were continued to influence the powers that be at the National Research Council-National Academy of Sciences in Washington, sponsors of the Commission, and were also to no avail, and my report to them concerning the work was never acknowledged. My hope of somehow reassuring the people of Hiroshima that their negative beliefs were unwarranted, that they could lead full and healthy lives, sadly had to be abandoned. There was just no way to get past the rigid belief structure of the medical profession that belief in early death could in any way hasten early death itself.

For many years, usually on the anniversary of the bombing of Hiroshima August 6, 1945, reports in the world press of how many thousands had died that year of A-bomb disease was cause of great sadness for me, for I felt so many could have been spared their final illness by simple encouragement and reassurance, that A-bomb disease was pure fiction, the result, at least in part, of a negative mindset. And further I was dismayed that the world medical community never questioned the phony diagnoses.

I have grieved through the years that the Hiroshima findings which I deemed so important were to be lost, and the fact that beliefs and attitudes could have a critical effect on human health and longevity, which was so apparent in Japan, could remain unseen and indeed overlooked.

Then HIV/AIDS came along in the mid-1980s, and I quickly recognized the analogy, the connection with what had occurred in Hiroshima. A sense of hopelessness and doom was developing in those infected with HIV quite similar to the feelings of those exposed to the atomic bomb in Japan. And I wondered, as I had in Hiroshima, whether this deep negativity in outlook was really warranted.

All epidemics in history have had natural survivors. Even in the worst ones, most who suffered the disease survived. There was no reason to believe in 1985 that HIV-infected people would be any different from those in past influenza, polio, or plague epidemics. There would be many survivors, many even who would have no manifestations of the disease whatever. The main difference with HIV/AIDS is the often prolonged latency period from initial infection with a virus to the disease called AIDS, which can extend to ten or more years. An article as late as 1988 speculated that it could be up to 30 years, admitting that they really could not know the answer to how many would survive.

How did the conventional wisdom go from "don't know" to the belief in 100% progression to AIDS? The media, incessantly and compulsively championing negativity, carry heavy responsibility. The AIDS activists loudly demanding attention in lobbying for money for research, shoot themselves in the foot by insisting on an always negative outcome for those testing positive for

HIV, their purpose being to move Congress to act when indeed they are convincing themselves of their own doom. It becomes more and more apparent that researchers, who give no credence to the power of doom, have encouraged the idea of the absolute progress to AIDS of the HIV-infected to increase their own self-importance and assure the continual inpouring of grants and funds. There may be no ill will on the part of the AIDS establishment, but rather an ignorance of its role in producing lethal doom in those with HIV.

The pervasive belief of friends and neighbors that those with HIV are certain to progress to AIDS is an additional powerful negative for those infected; their feelings of hopelessness are so often confirmed by everybody around them. Thus there is no source whatsoever of encouragement. Also, reports in the media are almost all negative, as well as official government reports by the Centers for Disease Control, world health organizations, and our National Institutes of Health. In addition, the consensus of AIDS researchers that either a cure or an effective vaccine against HIV/AIDS is so far off allows those presently infected no real hope. Even the currently widely used drugs against HIV have shown little promise that they can alter the disease or its eventual outcome. Drugs effective against manifestations of full-blown AIDS, due to the fact that the disease knocks out the immune system, can give temporary succor, but there is no treatment for AIDS itself.

If there are to be natural survivors of HIV, then those individuals would need no treatment whatsoever, and, in fact, treatment with currently used drugs would be contraindicated, since they all have toxicity and adverse side-effects which of themselves can cause severe illness. The drugs have wide use now because of the solid belief that all cases of HIV infection will lead to AIDS with 100% fatal outcome. If we knew or believed there would be many natural survivors, we would probably withhold such drugs until actual manifestations of the disease appeared. This is the only disease I know of where treatment with powerful drugs is begun several to many years prior to the actual onset of any illness, when there is still the possibility that AIDS may never develop.

I firmly believe that in the absence of the mindset of certain doom, there would be many more survivors of HIV than of those acquiring AIDS. Even if the negative set remains, I believe there will still be survivors. But how long do we have to wait to see? The proponents of doom will want to extend the period perhaps indefinitely. Instead, we should be searching, expectantly, for the natural survivors, long-term and in perfect health, who, I predict, will tell us that they maintained a positive attitude despite all the negative propaganda always surrounding them. Their stories could inspire and encourage others with HIV to alter their own negative attitudes and break out of their prisons of hopelessness. It is unknown how much good such positive information could do, but for people who have lived without hope for so long, the injection of even a little hope could do wonders for heart and soul. I'm convinced that the progression to AIDS could be reversed given a real and dynamic change in outlook. Considering the years that the process takes, there is plenty of time for a person to effect these changes. Let us hope that the natural suvivors will make themselves known in the coming years when they report with real confidence their positive experiences.

For those who have given up because of all the negativism surrounding their HIV infection, resentment against the injection of hope is also a possibility, especially if they have come to believe that the resolution of their plight rests in their own responsibility to pick themselves up and make the turnaround in attitude. They may simply not possess the strength, or the courage, or the will to change, after all the endless months and years of despair and hopelessness. It may seem easier to let the progression to AIDS happen than to summon enough strength to try another course. If so, the resentment against the intrusion of hope will be intense and many may reject the turnaround and eschew talk of hope and encouragement. Many sick people want to get well, but very few are willing to undergo the changes in themselves needed to gain that wellness, to search within themselves and really make the necessary corrections.

Hopelessness where HIV/AIDS is concerned also gives some kind of comfort to those who have already lost loved ones to AIDS. The idea of incurability and inexorability expunges any sense of self-responsibility in a universally fatal disease. It is fate striking down helpless victims. The idea that many HIV infected could be natural survivors if they could somehow overcome the pervasive and certain doom associated with the condition, would be very disturbing to those who watched their dear ones die of AIDS. Accordingly, they are vocal in their attacks on some health department pamphlets that refuse to state that HIV is eventually 100% fatal. Any loopholes of hope, they reason, will encourage young people to be more careless about safe sex. I understand their concern, but little do they realize that their actions are adding immeasurably to the AIDS death toll; their active support of hopelessness is just another manifestation of the awful state of doom that eats into the consciousness of all who are HIV-positive.

As terrible as the atomic bombing of Hiroshima was, activists for peace in the ensuing years have led a crusade to remind people all over the world of its horrific nature, including exaggeration of its late effects on health of the initial survivors, implying that even those who were alive after 10 or 20 years were still subject to dying from effects of the bomb. The message this gives to the survivors is the prospect that they still remain at risk. Thus the motivation of these peace groups to prevent the future use of nuclear weapons, a noble undertaking indeed, in actual fact does nothing to unseal the imagined fate of the fearful survivors. Similarly, with HIV presented as leading unequivocally to a fatal AIDS outcome, in a well-intended effort to frighten people to avoid unsafe sex, dirty needles, and infected blood derivatives, the threat so well publicized further confirms for those with HIV that they are surely doomed.

There now exists a great deal of confusion as to just how HIV infection progresses to the disease called AIDS. In fact, the HIV virus has not as yet been scientifically proven as the cause of AIDS, although the lay media seem to have assumed the connection as has the AIDS medical establishment directing most of the research. The victim's attitude, emotions, and morale appear to have no bearing on their research. In my own view, the progression of HIV infection to AIDS may depend in great measure on attitude as much as, or even more than, any other factors that may be involved.

To perhaps oversimplify, one can consider the following scenarios. Of course other factors are involved, but none could be more important than these:

> HIV infection, + treatment with powerful drugs, + an attitude of utter hopelessness over an extended period of time, and a gradual attrition with constant daily reminders of one's death sentence = AIDS.

> HIV infection, + an attitude of positivity and hope and self-confidence, + attention to good health maintenance, + cultivation of a positive self-image and self-knowledge, eschewing any treatment, = natural survival. Attitude is all-important, as in recovery and deliverance from any illness/disease situation, including, I daresay, even full-blown AIDS.

Corrections are in order. It is easy to sit back and say nothing, but somebody high up in the hierarchy of the AIDS establishment should step forward and say that he expects there will be natural survivors, in order to leave the door ajar for those diagnosed with HIV. Even that slight encouragement from some one in authority could do wonders for the morale of all those who are HIV-positive. I have watched and waited for years for this to happen, for someone from the NIH or from the CDC to refute the harbingers of doom, but in vain. Just saying, "I don't know", would have helped. Instead, the experts' silence has tended to seal the doom of those infected with the virus.

Perhaps support groups could be organized to effect deep changes in attitude, from certain negativity to really hopeful and realistic positivity. Encouragement in heavy and widespread doses could have done wonders in Hiroshima, but there simply wasn't any; in fact, just the opposite forces were at play. Now the situation with HIV/AIDS is strikingly and hauntingly similar — no encouragement and no hope, a situation which I believe is completely unwarranted, and surely subject to reversal.

Those who do reverse course and survive this scourge will stand as inspiration to all those infected. Only then will real answers regarding HIV/AIDS be forthcoming through careful investigations of differences in those survivors with eventual sufferers of AIDS. Such answers are simply not available to researchers convinced of HIV's eventual 100% mortality rate.

If the bridge between Hiroshima and HIV/AIDS could be clearly shown and gain acceptance by victims of the virus, the unrelieved sufferings and early death of the A-bomb survivors might at last find some meaning and requital - their sufferings would not have been in vain, but a gift to many others who were given no hope in another time, at another place.

CHAPTER IV

AIDS as Information Disease
(A Sequel to "Lessons from Hiroshima")[1]

George N. Hazlehurst

I. Background and Overview

My article on Hiroshima writen in 1993 was the result of many years of thought about AIDS. It reflected how deeply I felt about what I saw as a great injustice to so many people who happened to be HIV+ and who, in recent years, had been condemned to certain death by a government-sponsored powerful AIDS establishment. I knew their propaganda was false, especially equating AIDS with HIV, and recorded it in the Hiroshima article. Seeing the injustice and the lethal effect of the propaganda, I believed that my article might find acceptance in those affected by HIV/AIDS — the victims themselves and their loved ones and caregivers — offering hope and encouragement in a situation that thus far had been rife with utter despair and hopelessness. Distribution of the article to more than 200 HIV/AIDS support groups in early 1994, however, brought not a single response. It now seems essential, therefore, to enlarge upon the ideas there presented in the hope of fostering a more complete understanding.

---

[1]This essay has circulated in manuscript form, but is previously unpublished.

The mindset that HIV causes AIDS, and that AIDS is fatal, and that all of those with HIV will develop AIDS is the apparent consensus of the AIDS establishment and also of practically all of the media. How often we see it in print: "HIV, the virus that causes AIDS". The fact is that this has not been demonstrated by science as cause and effect. The evidence is at best only circumstantial, and mounting evidence by many scientists who oppose such an assumption of cause has been ignored and even pilloried by the main body of scientists who embrace the HIV=AIDS association. In alliance with the AIDS scientific establishment, our leading scientific journals also support the idea of HIV causing AIDS, and generally refuse to publish evidence to the contrary. Scientific consensus has coopted scientific proof.

During the summer of 1994, for the first time, information came to me that there are a significant number of scientists who disagree with the currently accepted HIV-causes-AIDS hypothesis, and who have been trying for several years against heavy odds to effect reappraisal of that hypothesis. I found this movement a very positive development, and I was amazed that I stumbled upon the group quite by accident. That I, so interested in the HIV/AIDS problem, had been quite unaware of any doctors or scientists opposed to the AIDS establishment, is a clear example of how our media have at the least neglected, and at the worst, suppressed any views that might oppose the majority view. I was amazed at how much information I could send for, and I am still attempting to absorb it all.

Here's an experiment that can't be performed because it would be extremely unethical and cruel: Tell a person that he or she is HIV+, even though it is untrue, and, with all the negative information now rampant in the media and accepted as "common knowledge" by almost everybody including that person's friends, relatives, and government, he or she will accept as fact that they are doomed to die of AIDS sooner or later. This individual will die of AIDS because he or she has accepted the prognosis as fact. There is little reason, in the present climate, for the person to believe otherwise, and he or she is doomed to die as scheduled.

Such an experiment is too dastardly even to imagine, isn't it? But I daresay, this very experiment may already have been unintentionally carried out. It is accepted by many that false positive HIV tests are not uncommon. Therefore, there must be some, perhaps many, who believed it when they were incorrectly told they were HIV+, and who have since been living with this nightmare. Some surely have proceeded to the end stage of AIDS. Some of these AIDS patients could be retested for HIV and found to be HIV-negative. It is the sense of hopelessness and discouragement itself which could be sufficient to eventually "deep-six" the immune system to a degree of non-functioning. The attitude of doom is lethal, not only in the case of HIV, but in any serious illness.

If belief in early death can cause early death, which seemed quite obvious in Hiroshima, then the HIV=AIDS belief fostered by the AIDS establishment has caused innumerable suffering and death, all needlessly. I am amazed to realize that so few people see what is happening. Worst of all, hardly anyone seems upset or even concerned. Those who feel doomed by it all have seemingly accepted their fate, even as they search about for medicines and elixirs to cure themselves. Usually they rely on establishment-hyped drugs like AZT, which have proven to be useless, are indeed toxic, and are deemed by some scientists to be actually causing some of the dire symptoms wrongly attributed to AIDS. Alternatively they seek out various medicinal herbs or other natural remedies still all the while waiting for a miracle cure or a vaccine to at last rescue them, which of course will never happen.

II. The Professionals' Plight

Let us examine the current medical system and how doctors are regulated in their medical practices, all to foster understanding of how an error from the most high can mean disaster to patients all over the world. First, all new ideas about treatment must come from the top, i.e., the ivory towers of medicine: the medical schools, the teaching hospitals, and the halls of power in the National Institutes of Health. Protocols for treatment of diseases are handed down via the myriad medical journals from on high, and end up finally in the medical practitioner's hands as "accepted medical treatment". They become the community standards of accepted practice, which are expected to be strictly adhered to. If they are not obeyed, and the doctor tries some different or original methods of handling a disease, he is subject to censure. Also, if he does not keep up with the latest protocols handed down from above, he is criticized by the system, so that he must spend any spare moments he might have in keeping up with the latest medical advances. It is impossible to keep up with the rapidly changing facets of therapeutics, yet he must try if he is to avoid censure or even malpractice litigation instigated by a disgruntled patient who can show that the doctor neglected to prescribe the latest treatments.

I bring up these points to show that any originality on the part of the doctor's treatments is actively discouraged by the system. He is to follow the protocol (the recipe book) without question, or he is in for trouble. The practice of medicine is, accordingly, not for anybody with a creative mind. He is not educated in order to create and advance the general knowledge. He is trained, rather, to follow orders passed down to him from the top of the medical hierarchy. Education and training are not the same thing. A technician is trained. A free-thinker is educated. The doctor is a technician; his freedom of thought is taken away. To see him in some artificial light, as humanitarian or savior, is a mistake. Today he has become a highly trained professional caught up in a narrowly mechanistic medical system, and his only hope to survive and prosper is to follow the strict rules provided from above.

What happens when a mistake is made at the top of the medical hierarchy? Disaster, widespread disaster, affecting the very lives of a great multitude of people. This is exactly what has happened in the HIV/AIDS fiasco: A gross mistake in the cause of AIDS attributed to a relatively innocuous virus. This misinformation took the usual course of passage down the medical chain of command to the doctors in the field. The word was that since AIDS is caused by a virus — an infection — it can only be controlled by drugs or the development of a vaccine to immunize against the virus. Protocols soon followed, and the doctors were finally in a position to offer treatment. The fact that the drugs were ineffective and had many toxic side effects made no difference. The treatment was set in stone, and was to be implemented by the doctors. Whether the toxicities killed some or many people was irrelevant. This was the accepted treatment, and was even prescribed for perfectly healthy individuals who had no signs of AIDS, but were HIV+.

Soon HIV+ and AIDS became interchangeable terms, and everybody who turned up antibody-positive was believed doomed to die (eventually) of AIDS. The term "People with AIDS" (PWA's) included all who were HIV+, even in the absence of AIDS.

When this HIV=AIDS=death became the commonly accepted reality a few years ago, I became suspicious that something very fishy was going on. Looking back on all the great historical epidemics, there were always survivors, natural survivors, and almost always far more who survived than did not survive. Yet here was a vicious epidemic among us in which no one who was infected was expected to survive. I kept waiting for someone high up in the medical hierarchy to say what should have been common knowledge among the researchers — that many, and probably the majority, of those infected would survive, all based on knowledge of past epidemics. Yet no one in the AIDS establishment has stepped forward to give this truthful information to the people. Instead, they remain silent, giving tacit support to the media's "no hope for HIV+" propaganda.

As in Hiroshima, where those exposed to the bombing believed they were doomed by A-bomb disease, so the HIV+ people feel doomed by AIDS. Why shouldn't they believe it when their government scientists, their doctors, their friends and relatives, and the media all believe it? The pressures to believe were so similar in both situations.

Now, more and more HIV+ individuals are long-term survivors. I wrote to one of the higher-ups at the NIH asking that someone there make a statement to the effect that they expect that there will be some natural survivors, and perhaps even express the hope that there might be many. I believed this was a reasonable suggestion and could offer real hope and encouragement to many who carry the viral antibodies. The response to my request skirted my concern and assured me that new treatments were in the offing. So any hope and encouragement, even if clearly warranted, is apparently a no-no to those in control of the NIH.

Who, if anybody, is at fault in this fiasco? I have no doubt that the researchers are sincere in their endeavors, and if by chance they see through the HIV/AIDS deception, they may be able to rationalize their silence in order to continue their work and their grants, their very livelihood. Also, the doctors involved with their patients are merely following orders given from on high, and are blameless. If their patients die from toxicity from drugs used to treat HIV/AIDS, they remain blameless, since they are merely following the protocols from the pharmaceutical giants which are sanctioned by the medical ivory towers. And those who originally blamed AIDS on HIV, although mistaken, were under intense pressure to produce results and could have acted in good faith. It is simply an unfortunate chain of events that has led to the current tragedy of AIDS.

Does anybody benefit from this status quo? Yes, lots and lots of people. Consider just how many people the war on AIDS employs. It's a huge army, supported almost entirely by us as taxpayers or as donors to innumerable AIDS-related charities. It has become a multibillion dollar industry, whose tentacles extend into every community. The fear of HIV/AIDS has become world-wide.

III. True Believers and the Cult of Doom

To alter the situation, we must get rid of the false belief. But first we must go back to find the origin of the false belief, and that began with some very careless research that led to the historic announcement in 1984 by the government that the "probable cause of AIDS" had been found, and that was a retrovirus named HTLV-III (later re-named HIV). This was soon followed by a test developed to find antibodies to the virus, and ever since it was decided that anyone who tests positive for HIV is doomed to develop AIDS and die. The belief in fatal outcome has become stronger and stronger over the years.

Now something did cause the outbreak of AIDS in the gay community, but it wasn't HIV, and nobody could be sure just what it was. But, convinced that HIV was the cause, the AIDS establishment has never pursued the real cause. The ideas of alternate causes presented by researchers who understand the false basis of the HIV cause are completely ignored by the AIDS establishment, which has become, mainly through billions in government funding, a huge political power that will tolerate no interference.

What's happened to the HIV/AIDS victims? Well, they've formed a huge cult of true believers in their own doom, and they too will permit no interference in this mindset. They sympathize with and support one another with religious fervor, feeling they have finally discovered the meaning and purpose of their lives, and write often with great enthusiasm on the subject of their death and dying. They have accepted the "facts" and have completely accommodated to their own death sentence.

There does seem to be a glorification of HIV/AIDS, even as a magnet of compassion and a celebrity life — a meaning and purpose for lives that may have lacked such qualities before being infected and pitied, and even taking on heroic proportions as kinds of martyrs. Here were lives perhaps lacking in self-esteem suddenly in the forefront of an historic meaning, victims of the great AIDS epidemic of the latter part of the 20th century.

Can anything be done for the people who believe they are doomed to die of AIDS because they are HIV+ ? The belief is firm and continuously strengthened by daily negative propaganda bombarding them on all sides. How then is it possible to effect a reversal in attitude, in thinking, and to instill certain knowledge that they can become well, or, if well, can stay well?

It would require, I think, intensive reprogramming of the human bio- computer. Just how difficult that might be is seen in efforts to deprogram individuals caught up in the various religious cults. As in the cults, the people who are HIV+ have been brainwashed, and they are virtually trapped in belief systems that guarantee a fatal outcome.

It is not, then, just a simple matter of telling these people that the whole AIDS thing was a mistake, that they're really not destined to get AIDS, not to worry. This was the theme of my Hiroshima article, that all that was needed was an injection of hope and encouragement, which I soon discovered was simply not so. These people need to be deprogrammed if they are to recover, and that will require first a willingness on their part even to undergo such a program and an intensive effort by some organized competent and capable entity to carry out the deprogramming. The probability that such a plan could succeed is far from certain, especially in the presence of continuing negative propaganda by the establishment and the continuing attraction of the cult-like mass of HIV+ true believers in certain death.

How to explain resistance to rescue, when the rescuee doesn't understand it himself? How can he be saved? It's the horse to water dilemma. Perhaps rescue is impossible without drastic change in thinking, unless there is an ocean shift in thinking so powerful that the resister can't help but be swept up in the mass movement. There is the unlikely possibility that someone in authority could announce that the HIV thing was all a mistake. The trouble is, there is no person with that much authority, and individuals in command of the HIV-AIDS establishment, even if they see the truth and want to help correct the error, are far too weak to effect any change in course. They are all trapped in the gargantuan propaganda mill of their own making and are helpless to escape it. Perhaps a president, a senator, a congressman? Is there one of such stature? Maybe somebody in the media could be heard, but the commentators and columnists of today seem without stature, their words of no real import or impact, apparently deathly afraid of offending their employers.

Although there may be no real hope for change or correction in the short haul, there probably is hope in the long run, which may be the real reason for this writing. To get to those who do see the error and so want to contribute to its correction, it may be possible that the insights presented here might be helpful in the future in the eventual resolution of this very tricky and complicated problem. Valuable knowledge of human behavior may be the end result and give a positive twist to what appears now to be a great human tragedy. When it becomes evident, moreover, that one's beliefs can literally kill one, this will be a great step forward in understanding health and disease. That it may take many more deaths to show this seems unfortunate, but is apparently essential to prove the case.

We must continue to focus on rescue: How to direct people away from this belief in their inevitable doom from HIV towards the realization that they have within them the power to continue living as well. How to wake up the true believer in his own doom. There appears to be no easy, gentle way.

Being misled can be subtle,insidious, and almost imperceptible, an unseen force at play that can easily brainwash most people.

It can be a charismatic leader, followed by believers, or consensus reality fueled by huge propaganda machines professing: This is truth; this is the cause of AIDS. To reverse such beliefs, by now so deeply ingrained, meets fierce resistance. There is also the AIDS activists' resistance to AIDS being caused by factors other than HIV, and insistence on powerful drugs even if untested and dangerous. Nobody speaks of getting well or staying well, so solid is the certainty of death in these people.

So what do you do? The constant hammering of the truth that HIV does not cause AIDS must be aimed at those who are HIV+ if change is to occur. It is they who must see the truth and rebel against the AIDS establishment, the ones who keep pushing the deadly propaganda. We're quite used to seeing government officials and scientists and doctors as authority figures, but all this has to change, as these once respected individuals have become the agents of death when it comes to HIV/AIDS.

IV. Support Groups to Die For; Ways to Resist the Doomsayers

A real problem and obstacle to helping sick people is that humans can accommodate and adjust all too quickly to chronic illness. The person actually gets used to being sick, accepts the prognosis given by the doctor, and if death is in the prospect, that too is accepted as a given. This process takes place usually over many months, but once this mindset is in place, it seems simply not possible to reverse it. If I, as a physician, at this point of complete accommodation, try to intervene and encourage the person to get well, I am met with total resistance. I believe this is the case with all those who are HIV+ and have reached a point of accommodation with their "illness", even though in all physical measures they are perfectly well people.

What happens to the true believers in their own certain death from AIDS? They form support groups which seem to be designed to offer moral support to their members, to help them accommodate to the inevitable outcome of a 100% fatal disease. Those in charge of such groups, whether carrying the HIV antibodies or healthy volunteers, must feel great satisfaction in doing such good deeds in behalf of those doomed to die of AIDS. These well-meaning support groups are of course quite unaware that they are hastening these people's eventual demise by helping their accommodation to their "fatal illness".

To resist the doomsayers, solutions reside with the American people who always have it within their power to effect change, completely outside prevailing negative forces.

Here are four such possibilities:

1. Insist that everybody be tested for the HIV virus. Of course this is not going to happen, but the results could be astonishing if it were found that many people of all ages are HIV+. An accurate epidemiologic study of HIV has not been possible because of legal and social restrictions on testing. If everybody were tested, it might well indicate that HIV is a common virus widespread in the general population, probably even including some prominent members of the AIDS establishment.

2. Decline being tested for HIV. Since the sense of certain doom is the main result of a positive test, this lethal mindset could be eliminated. If the test is positive, the experts say you're doomed, so why risk taking on such a bleak status?

3. Is HIV contagious? It is difficult to believe, but even this question has not been fully answered. As there is no scientific evidence, anyway, that HIV causes AIDS, the question of how

HIV is transmitted becomes moot, and since there is no "AIDS virus", this is all the more reason to refuse testing. Above all, refuse treatment with so-called antiviral drugs, no matter what the doctors tell you.

It should be made clear that drugs used to treat illness caused by a broken immune system are not the object of criticism. It is the antiviral drugs that are to be condemned because, not only are they very toxic, but they are useless against an entirely fictional AIDS virus.

4. Despite the overwhelming propaganda by the AIDS industry, there exist individuals who are long-term HIV+ survivors who are able to discount the pervasive negatives all about them and get on with their lives. It is hard to imagine what kind of person could survive so devastating a death sentence. It would have to be someone very special, a person of great strength of character and moral substance. That there are such people out there, I know for sure, because I have found one such person who has been HIV+ for 17 years, is in perfect health, and knows that he will so remain. He knows that attitude is all-important, and refuses to accept the onslaught of negatives that bombard us constantly. To borrow from a somewhat famous statement: It's the attitude, stupid.

A definite hope lies in the possibility that long-term survivors of the HIV scare may come together and provide leadership within the AIDS activist community toward pushing a campaign for the return to health and wellbeing for those who are HIV+, this to replace the policy of progression to certain death sanctioned by the AIDS establishment. Such a movement within that community could do wonders, and might make the seemingly onerous task of massive deprogramming unnecessary. To so effect a sudden paradigm shift is a definite possibility, and it could be brought about completely separate from the powerful and unbending AIDS orthodoxy.

V. Truth, Belief, and Information Disease

What is truth? What is right and what is wrong? We would like to turn to the prophets for answers. Hard science attracts us mightily because it is so certain in its truths. 2+2=4. But what we are to believe in other kinds of information is uncertain. So we look for answers to sticky questions by public opinion polls, which now take the place of seeking out the prophets that no longer exist for us. Simply put, if most people believe something to be true, or right, or wrong, then that something must be true or right or wrong. The beliefs of the majority become our truths. Is this not democracy's way?

In our current era of massive information cast at us on a daily schedule, we are overwhelmed and completely helpless to process all the input to decide which is true and which is not. The onslaught is so overpowering that our minds seem to accept as true far more than they should. It amounts to brainwashing on a grand scale, and influential far beyond anything we may imagine. The advertising industry alone has honed its skills at persuasion to ever finer techniques, making it impossible for the consumer to make rational choices. Misinformation therefore becomes the norm, and the whole culture becomes permeated with a predominance of lies, and truth becomes more and more a stranger to us all.

Advertising we may accept as false and believe that's no big deal, simply adding to the general level of misinformation. But other forms of misinformation can do far greater damage than we imagine, and there are threats that reach us every day via the media, and are in the form of warnings about our health and even our very survival. We've seen it all, and what are we to do? One day it's things we eat that are bad for us; the next day it's not true, it's other things that are bad for us. Over and over it happens. And everything we can imagine is blamed for cancer, at one time or another, and then an opposite opinion appears. Many medical "facts" that we've been led to accept as truth have never been proven.

All illnesses contain elements of information disease. Cancer has had a very bad press for a very long time, and the diagnosis carries with it a dread of probable doom. How do the victims overcome this negative mindset and somehow bring about spontaneous healing, which we know is possible, when an impenetrable wall of complete discouragement is erected around them?

Every disease carries its own negative information, always accepted and believed by the one who is ill. Even the common cold has its set parameters as to kinds and duration of symptoms, to be expected, and therefore to be experienced. Each illness lives up to the common knowledge that we hold of it, and it turns out that we get exactly what we expect of it.

Primitive peoples, in their inherent wisdom, would recognize a hex when they saw one, and would have prescribed methods to deal with such things, perhaps through healing rituals performed by a shaman, a witch doctor, a medicine man, or an exorcist. Our culture, however, is far too civilized, educated, and sophisticated to believe in the casting of spells, and when we are all hexed by the AIDS industry's hoax, we are helpless to act because we have no remedies in place to deal with such phenomena.

VI. A Plea for Cooperation and Reappraisal

There are deep concerns as to what might happen if and when the truth emerges. It would be a terrible blow to biomedical science, with reputations in ruins and means of making a living threatened, along with fear of disgrace and humiliation — a mortal blow to science and medicine generally. And it will spell devastation to HIV+ people who truly believe in their inevitable death. Relief at rescue? Surprise! — just the opposite. Complete resistance. They will go on and die anyway, unless some kind of deprogramming can be devised to save them.

The result of truth finally realized will be complete pandemonium. Can anything be done to avert such disaster? Instead of the contention between the AIDS establishment and its critics now present, could the proponents on each side somehow come together and work out some kind of face-saving plan? It could begin by both sides cutting out the belligerent behavior, discontinue spouting mean things about one another, and instead encourage open debate in order for the truth to emerge. If errors have been made, they must be uncovered and admitted to. Suppression of divergent views must halt. All parties should be working together to solve the AIDS crisis.

A good beginning might be the universal adoption of the very reasonable request for reappraisal of the HIV-AIDS hypothesis requested during the past few years by a group who believe we're on the wrong track, and who have been ignored by the AIDS establishment. The work of an independent investigating body should be supported by all to flush out the truth about what is the true cause of AIDS. All beliefs and opinions on the subject must give way to findings of real knowledge, which is the way science is supposed to work. A hypothesis is not truth, and surely does not become truth just because a majority of scientists believe it. Consensus reality is not reality, and only prevents our finding and seeing reality.

The powerful propaganda machine run by the AIDS establishment and disseminated by the media must be halted, and above all, the patent lie that AIDS is caused by the HIV virus has to be retracted. Even after 10 years of intense research, the connection between HIV and AIDS remains unproven, and on that basis alone, the hypothesis should be discarded, especially when other causes promulgated by researchers outside the AIDS establishment make far more sense. To discard 10 years of work and go back to square one may seem hard to do, but it must be done. And not with regret and continued rancor, but with humility and cooperation by all concerned parties.

If the original epidemic of AIDS in the early 80's was related to overuse of illegal or recreational drugs, and of prescription drugs for frequently recurring infections related to promiscuous life styles in the gay community, which many researchers believe to be the case, that could be shown to be true through careful study. Thus far such an avenue has been prohibited by the virus-hunter powers in the government who go to extreme lengths to protect the HIV-causes-AIDS hypothesis.

My own conviction that AIDS has become an information disease, caused by the doomsaying constantly spewed out from the AIDS establishment since 1985, could also be demonstrated by careful study and participation by all concerned, especially those suffering from AIDS or who are HIV+. For example, a survey could be developed asking such questions as: "What effect has the heavy and continuing propaganda of doom had on you personally? What effect on your outlook, on your attitude? Do you believe what you hear about HIV causing AIDS? Why do you so believe?"

I think the position of the fully indoctrinated victim is completely understandable and quite legitimate. They respond to doubts about the HIV=AIDS hypothesis with, "How could everybody be so wrong? The media, the government scientists, the CDC, the NIH, the doctors everywhere, all the medical journals, the medical textbooks, the drug publications, in addition to all the AIDS support groups, all the publications put out by large AIDS organizations, in addition to friends and family — all believe that HIV=AIDS=death. How can I believe it's not true?"

Enter information disease, perhaps better named "misinformation" disease, a plague that has engulfed the whole world.

VII. Remaining Questions, a Quest for Clarity, and the End of Doom

In conclusion, a few loose ends cry for attention. Most important, nobody sees that the power of doom can cause the immune system to crash, and everybody believes that AIDS is caused by a virus. The combination of these two mental states (one of not-seeing and one of over-believing) makes the emergence of truth extremely difficult.

There are several main reasons why the immune system can wear itself out and eventually fail. Often overlooked is the fact that mental depression can affect immunity, and it is quite likely that depressed immunity is a factor in any serious illness, and could indeed be the chief factor.

I don't think people realize how devastating the stigma of HIV positivity has become. Loss of jobs, of insurance, thoughts of suicide and attempts thereat, financial ruin, rejection and alienation — all are enough to drive anyone into a state of hopeless depression, and all in addition to the prospect of early and horrible death practically guaranteed by the experts. Aside from this doom mindset, those carrying HIV antibodies are barred from many activities, such as travel abroad, and in at least one country they are incarcerated to prevent the "epidemic" from spreading. Blood banks and their directors have been sued and prosecuted for allowing "infected" blood to be distributed, and now all blood for transfusion has to be tested at enormous expense. There is even talk of discharging HIV+ members of our Armed Forces.

The habit of doctors and medical scientists to discount and ignore the sick person's attitude, his hopes, his despair, his outlook builds up a huge blind spot covering the most important aspect of his being. The distinct possibility that AIDS can be caused by the person's certain belief that he is doomed to die of AIDS, as is the case with those who find they are HIV+, is surely present. Why is it ignored?

The plights of HIV in children and expectant mothers and the HIV-infected masses in subSaharan Africa beg for clarification. All are imbued with the mindset of doom, the Africans by constant propaganda broadcast by the World Health Organization. All peoples have feelings, and there's no reason why condemned Africans should react any differently. Of course they believe it when the authorities tell them they are doomed.

As for the babies who are infected with HIV in utero, the doctors prescribe the useless but toxic drugs to expectant mothers and babies alike. Babies are far more sensitive and intelligent than we imagine, and they do absorb emotion like a sponge, no matter how young. Parents who believe in their own doom as well as the doom of their infected babies and older children can't help but transfer that negative emotion to the little ones. Those babies also can't help but feel the deprivation of love from parents who are incapable of bestowing lifesaving love upon a small child that they know is slated for early death.

The AIDS establishment has put great stock in the high correlation of AIDS with the presence of HIV antibodies. This is partially contrived, since if AIDS is present in the absence of HIV antibodies, the scientists label it as a separate disease. The main reason for correlation, however, is that the certain doom associated with HIV positivity does of itself cause eventual AIDS. In that case, a virtually complete correlation would be expected. If you scare someone to death, of course there is a correlation between the scare and the death. It doesn't take a highly placed scientist to see that. Yet when it comes to HIV causing AIDS by sheer terror, that same scientist is struck blind.

The lengthy latent period from the positive HIV antibody test to the development of AIDS has been set at about 10 years, which can give a perfectly healthy individual plenty of time to absorb and react to the constant deadly propaganda. He may bravely try to carry on, but eventually the death sentence can penetrate any armoring he may erect to protect himself and through gradual attrition he will eventually succumb.

That prolonged stretch from doom to death is so unusual that it should have attracted our suspicions early on. It can only be explained by the heavy propaganda designed to protect the HIV-causes-AIDS hypothesis. When some HIV+'s kept surviving longer and longer, the powers at the NIH simply extended the "incubation period", and they can continue to extend it, keeping the fear alive for years to come.

In summary, the series of events that have led to the current AIDS crisis are easy to trace — a tragedy of errors and misconceptions and a careless acceptance of sloppy science by experts and general public alike.

Mistake #1: The outbreak of AIDS in the gay community blamed on a virus, as other possible causes were virtually ignored. There has never been any proof of AIDS being caused by an infectious agent.

Mistake #2: Discovery of the HIV virus, which was arbitrarily assigned the cause of AIDS without any confirmation whatsoever by other scientists.

Mistake #3: A test devised to detect antibodies to HIV. Now the "cause" of AIDS could be detected and confirmed, and this was the start of the disease of doom. Everybody who tested positive was destined to get AIDS and, of course, die. No exceptions. Without doubt the most effective terrorist campaign in history, with no end to its destruction in sight.

Unless ... Unless we can all wake up and see what is happening. And then get together and do something about it. The hope must remain that those doomed may yet be salvaged.

CHAPTER V

The Psychohistorical Origins of AIDS:
An Interview with Casper Schmidt[1]

Ian Young

> *"What is disease? It is false reasoning.... I will say to the patient, 'You have built the disease yourself, in your sleep of ignorance.' ... I know that the bottom of these phenomena is a lie in the beginning and started by a liar till it was received as true; then the phenomenon is called disease."*
>
> — Phineas P. Quimby, c. 1860

I first heard of Casper Schmidt in the late Eighties, when I was compiling the bibliography of alternative approaches to AIDS that became *The AIDS Dissidents.* My friend and fellow researcher John Lauritsen sent me an article entitled "The Group-Fantasy Origins of AIDS", which *The Journal of Psychohistory* had published a few years earlier in its Summer 1984 issue. That paper, published in the year the official line on AIDS was pronounced, represented one of the earliest — and most intriguing — dissenting views about the epidemic. There, Dr. Casper Schmidt, a gay psychoanalyst, considered AIDS in the light of certain unconscious American group-fantasies, and compared it to a number of "hysterical epidemics" in recent history.

---

[1]This interview has not previously been published.

Schmidt was one of the first to explore the psychosocial background to the health crisis, maintaining that the strident political attacks on gays that persisted throughout the Seventies had contributed to a shame-based, sacrificial group psychology among gay men, which in turn led to "an epidemic of depression with psychogenically-reduced cell-mediated immunity". Authorities and the media participated in the general trance state.

A medical doctor with a psychoanalytic practice in New York, Schmidt also served as Associate Director of The Institute of Psychohistory. Born in South Africa, where he had published several books of poetry in Afrikaans, he spent two years working as a physician in the Black township of Soweto before moving to the U.S. in 1975 to train as a psychiatrist, specializing in adolescent, child and infant psychology. In New York, he was also known as an enthusiastic member of the AIDS activist group ACT UP.

I arranged to meet Casper Schmidt on a sunny, blustery morning in November of 1992, in a diner on Broadway. He struck me as a good-natured man in his forties, with a penetrating intelligence that was based on keen powers of observation. After breakfast, we walked a few blocks to his psychiatric consulting rooms overlooking Riverside Park on Manhattan's Upper West Side.

I began our interview by asking about psychohistory. Referring to Lloyd deMause's definition of psychohistory as "the science of historical motivation", Casper went on to distinguish three types of psychohistory: psychobiography (mostly of leaders and other prominent individuals); the history of childhood — the different ways children have been treated historically, and the results; and group psychology in its political context. He noted that ninety percent of current psychohistory is psychobiography, which he said he regarded as being to some degree a defense against childhood and group psychohistory. I asked him why.

CS: "Because the fantasies that come together in political life reach to such a profound level of the unconscious and are so disturbing and upsetting that most people find them extremely difficult to deal with. For example, if you say, 'We want to sacrifice the leader', that simple sentence — for which we have such ample evidence — provokes immoderate amounts of anxiety because it confronts them with the deepest levels of unconscious motivation."

IY: "So the whole fantasy of the sacrifice of a Sacred King like Kennedy throws them into a tizzy and they posit the idea of a lone, crazy person who has nothing to do with the rest of us and is cut off from us by mental disturbance and so on."

CS: "The one thing that people can tolerate is to enact the fantasies on the historical stage — if they can project the blame onto somebody or other. Looking at this in a rational, scientific way seems to most people like the most difficult thing on earth."

Six years after Schmidt's arrival in America, the AIDS crisis began. Schmidt began to investigate the syndrome after one of his patients had a lover who had fallen ill:

CS: "The more I read, the more puzzling and the more profoundly disturbing it became. Because it made no sense. At that point, everybody was conceptualizing AIDS as an infectious disease which was spread by sexual contact. And as I was looking through the evidence, it became more and more clear to me that this epidemic was not behaving like an infectious disease at all."

IY: "This would be before the pronouncement of the official HIV idea."

CS: "Yes, this was in 1983, about a year before HIV [was publicized]. But already, people were speaking about a virus in our bloodstream, which was a phrase Reagan would use throughout his term in office. Yet even at that stage, the idea was that this was something spread sexually and through drug use."

The ideas about "safe sex" that were evolving even then in the gay community Schmidt described as "an apotropaic ritual" designed to ward off the dangers of sexual contamination:

CS: "The further I read about this, the less sense it made. Infectious epidemics do not follow fault lines that are cultural or sociological, which is what we find in this epidemic. You do not find any infectious epidemic in history that selectively infects a group designated on a basis of cultural factors."

I asked about the European diseases (like smallpox) that devastated the Native peoples of the Americas:

CS: "There you have quite a different situation. Europeans had, through centuries of contact with certain diseases, built up what is called herd immunity. All those people who were susceptible to these diseases died out through the centuries. Everyone who remained had immunity. When these same diseases were transferred to a new population, you had an abbreviated replay of what had happened in Europe — all over the place, all at once, with devastating results. This is typical of infectious epidemics.

"Hepatitis B is an infectious disease spread through a virus, through sexual contact, contact with blood and other intimate contact. Hepatitis B is somewhat restricted to certain groups, particularly gay men, because of the upsurge of sexual contacts during the Seventies, in bathhouses and so on. However, it was not totally restricted to those people, so that any physician, for example, who came into contact with the virus was at risk. And it spreads whenever there is sexual contact — regardless of sexual orientation.

"That's the difference between an infectious disease and what you have in AIDS, where the spread is virtually entirely according to cultural parameters. In the beginning, it was with gay men, and as the Reagan administration [established itself in] power, with drug addicts. And those were the two main scapegoat groups, and a few smaller groups that may have had unconscious identifications with us when you had unconscious fantasies of poisoned blood, which were rampant during the Reagan/Bush years."

I asked about hemophiliacs, and Schmidt pointed out that hemophiliacs have incredible numbers of blood transfusions, causing a phenomenon called tolerance, which is very similar to AIDS.

IY: "Hemophiliacs have always died at a great rate."

CS: "Even more importantly, there is an enormous literature on the psychology of hemophilia. All the male children with hemophilia are subjected to the most restrictive regimen, which inhibits their ability to express aggression — something which I think is necessary for this kind of syndrome to develop. This is a factor which they share with drug addicts and gay men. All these groups of people had in earlier life a curtailment of their right to express their aggression in an unfettered way. That is one of the risk factors for this syndrome."

IY: "How does this aggression factor pertain to gay men?"

CS: "A drive seeks to be expressed. It has no concern whether outwards or inwards. When the expression of this drive is curtailed for whatever reason, the drive is often turned inwards and expressed against the self, giving rise to psychosomatic disorders, actual physiological disturbances. That is what happens in AIDS. For example, it has become obvious that the people with AIDS who are least inhibited in their expression of aggression, and who pursue their own well-being with the least amount of curtailment, do best. They survive the longest — regardless of where they are in the syndrome. Those who do not express their aggression, their assertiveness, their right to exist, to the same extent, seem to come down with the syndrome in a rapid, usually fatal way."

IY: "You're talking here about characteristics of long-term survivors — what Michael Callen was looking at in his book *Surviving AIDS*?"

CS: "Yes. These are the people who are not afraid to get angry and to express their anger. These are people who demand and are not afraid of expressing their demands."

IY: "Bernie Siegel, in *Love, Medicine and Miracles*, says the same about cancer patients."

CS: "One hundred percent identical. When people do not express these basic drives, they are expressed instead as stress. Both AIDS and cancer patients feel abnormal stressors and feelings of helplessness. As a result, their bodies secrete a substance known as cortisol. Cancer patients show an enormous increase in cortisol and a lowering of their DHEAS levels, the same as in AIDS. Until two years ago, nobody had been able to figure out the function of the DHEAS, which is by far the most voluminous of all the steroid hormones in the body. The key factor in terms of both cancer patients and PWAs is that they feel great stress and helplessness. And instead of expressing their needs outwardly, they turn inward and over-secrete cortisol, which paralyzes their immune systems."

IY: "You see a sequence of events in the body that leads to the drop in T-cells that accompanies AIDS."

CS: "That's right. Pneumocystis carinii, for example (a serious illness of PWAs) is fought by T-cells producing gamma-interferon. If you have normal T-cells, the chance of developing pneumocystis is extremely low."

IY: "What part do you think venereal diseases play in the development of AIDS?"

CS: "Very little actually. I think they're mostly a marker for something else. The penumbral syndrome surrounding AIDS started in the mid-Seventies and showed itself in the enormous increase of venereal diseases and what was then called Gay Bowel Syndrome.... Everybody thinks that amoebiasis was driven by these wicked amoebas. In fact, I think a more accurate interpretation would be that the reduction in cellular immunity permitted amoebas to grow. The enormous incidence of venereal disease during the Seventies was a marker for people with a psychological vulnerability to the group psychology, and who responded to it with numerous anonymous sexual contacts, which increased the transmission of genuine venereal diseases — including syphilis, which is not so easy to treat as people think!"

Schmidt said he regarded the binge of anonymous gay sex that began in the Seventies as intimately related to the psychology of ostensibly heterosexual men, and also as deeply enmeshed with gay men's guilt feelings, tension and anger, which, deprived of any other outlet, tended to be repressed into the body. This somatization caused blocked emotions and profound biophysical changes. One of the most important of these has been the continuous simulation of a "fight or flight" syndrome.

The "fight or flight" syndrome occurs at times of increased stress and is accompanied by, among other things, temporary immune suppression and raised levels of adrenalin, endorphins and cortisol. Ordinarily, this syndrome should occur in humans only occasionally, in instances of danger. If it becomes, instead, a condition of life, cortisol levels become perpetually elevated. I asked Schmidt about the role of cortisol levels in AIDS.

CS: "All the work on cortisol levels in AIDS was done in 1988 but not published until 1992 because the researcher, Joseph Malone of the U.S. Marine Corps, working at the San Diego Naval Hospital, thought it was so far out of whack with the mainstream that there was no point in trying to publish it. Only in 1992 did he publish it. Malone was the pioneer who first looked at cortisol levels in AIDS. Since then, it's been confirmed that from day one in the spectrum of AIDS diseases, you have an overproduction of cortisol. That becomes consistently higher as the syndrome progresses and by the end of the syndrome, people overproduce cortisol in enormous amounts, like cancer patients."

Schmidt explained that the balance of cortisol and DHEAS affect interleukin-2 and gamma-interferon levels in the body. Interleukin-2 is the T-cell growth factor, which all T-helper lymphocytes need in order to exist. Research has shown that if they are deprived of Interleukin-2 for six to twelve hours, they undergo changes, called apoptosis, which result in T-cell destruction. So overproduction of cortisol, and a lack of Interleukin-2, can result in the killing of lymphocytes — both indirectly (by depriving them of growth factor) and directly (through the toxic effects of cortisol itself).

CS: "Everyone who proceeds to AIDS has lowered levels of DHEAS. That's the key pathogenetic mechanism, I think, in the entire syndrome. This is corroborated by the fact that PWAs have an overactivity of B-cells. A message goes out to the B-cells, 'Produce antibodies! Produce antibodies!' And they produce antibodies to everything they've been exposed to in the past, regardless of whether it's a current problem. And the B-cells go haywire, producing enormous amounts of antibodies.

"All of this dovetails with the work done with DHEAS. The guy who is most intimately connected with this and who discovered how this works is Raymond A. Daynes at the University of Utah."

IY: "This mechanism is a result of what kind of stresses?"

CS: "All the details haven't been worked out, but we do know several things. In Philadelphia in the Sixties, they found that if you put animals in a situation they can't escape from, and give them electric shocks, they try to escape for a certain time, but when they realize they can't escape, they lie down and tolerate the shocks, whimpering and moaning. If you open the gates of their cage, they behave as if they're still prisoners. They develop learned helplessness.

"All you need to do is to drag them out of the cage, and then they learn very quickly. Stephen Maier at the University of Colorado has worked out the physiology of this; there are biochemical reactions in the endorphin system which affect lymphocytes directly. Also, there are changes in the hypothalamus which cause the secretion of cortisol. Any kind of restraint, learned helplessness, or belief that people can have no impact on their situation, causes these changes.

"When individuals don't feel they can influence political life, if you have a conservative swing, with Reagan coming the White House, promulgating the fantasies of the far Right, saying that homosexuals are bad because they are destroying the family life of America and they should die, that is the kind of thing which creates inescapable stress, giving rise to feelings of helplessness. People don't know what to do, they don't have anything they can do. With the exception of ACT UP. That's where ACT UP comes in, because there, people are not helpless! They can release their feelings and express them. Which is why most of the people in ACT UP don't easily die from AIDS. We have an enormous and beautiful track record of people surviving much better. Expressing their rage is what saves them!"

I asked about HIV, the retrovirus that has been pronounced the official "cause" of AIDS.

CS: "I was never impressed with HIV as the cause of the syndrome, for various reasons. Most important, a virus like this does not remain confined to cultural categories. I thought there must be some other explanation for this. Indeed there is: epidemic hysteria. When you have people low down on the totem pole of power: women, prisoners, children, homeless people, people who feel powerless, those are the people who do not have an avenue to express their rage, they turn this inward and become ill with epidemic hysteria. AIDS is a clear case of epidemic hysteria.

"HIV, a relatively weak virus, belongs to the family of retroviruses. Characteristically, the retroviruses do not kill cells, they cause them to proliferate. So from the word go, when people said this weak virus kills the T-cells, it didn't make sense to me. All the evidence was against it. Plus — and this is where the theoretical sine qua non arises, that most people are trying to ignore, because they are all in a trance — there are many people who have the syndrome without any evidence for the virus."

Though Casper Schmidt was one of the first to question the role of HIV, he pointed out that the first to publish his skepticism was a French scientist by the name of Georges Matté. But it is Dr. Peter Duesberg, he said, who has made the most cogent arguments.

CS: "A man in Montreal called Hugo Soudeyns discovered that HIV has two receptors for cortisol. This makes a lot of sense because these receptors allow cortisol to have an effect on the virus; cortisol may be necessary for its growth. This was discovered by people in Robert Gallo's lab in 1986! They showed that cortisol stimulates the growth of HIV in the test-tube. So this explains the fit between incidence of the virus and the syndrome."

IY: "Yet there are people with HIV antibodies who are not sick."

CS: "Yes. If you don't have all the psychological factors that go into making the syndrome, you can have the virus and it will have little effect — similar to cytomegalovirus or some of the herpes viruses. You can have these viruses floating around in your body all your life without ever becoming sick from them. Ninety percent of gay men have cytomegalovirus. But only when your immune system is drastically disempowered do you get sick."

We talked about the role of the AIDS crisis in changing the status of gays in America.

CS: "Whenever people have become part of the group psychology of the mainstream, they have always entered through a period of sacrifice. The Jews in Europe went through an extended period of sacrifice before they were accepted. My reading of the AIDS crisis is that it is really part of the assimilation of gays into the political life of the country as a whole. And I think all of this started in the late Forties with the end of Isolationism and the assumption of America as the dominating power of the world. This gave Americans incredible amounts of hubris!

"Then, I think Kinsey was extremely important. Kinsey published [his first report on human sexuality] in the late Forties and caused an upheaval in this country. For the first time in the history of the world you had an accurate, statistical representation of what people actually did sexually. Everybody was driven insane because their cherished group-fantasies were completely demolished in two volumes! So immediately you had a reaction, which was McCarthyism. The cover was blown off the defenses. Those people who had strong homoerotic fantasies and couldn't deal with them were driven totally insane by Kinsey."

IY: "Like Hoover and McCarthy!"

CS: "Of course! People who were deepest in the closet and were most repressed. We were suddenly a great power 'on the world stage' and all our secrets were being published in books! This gave rise on the one hand to McCarthyism and all the paranoia it entailed. But on the other hand, you have the feeling that we can tolerate much more than before. So Frank Kameny and the Mattachine Society and the Daughters of Bilitis were all more advanced people, more in touch with the group fantasy of tolerance and openness. By the late Fifties came Women's Liberation, the Men's Movement, the Gay Movement. Then came the conservative clampdown of the late Seventies.

"I think that the end result of all of this will be that you will have virtually no overt homophobia or severe discrimination against gays in the future. But there will always be pockets of homophobia because abused children need to project their bad feelings somewhere. There will always be fag-bashers among boys who have been severely treated — and despised — by their fathers. In time, this too will change. Because America has become the first society to say that child abuse is unacceptable! I foresee a society which is relatively peaceful ... after the epidemic is over.

"Most epidemics are symmetrical. They rise and fall in a curve. Since the AIDS epidemic peaked for gay men in 1988, we can expect the epidemic to be over for gay men by 1996-7. What the Centers for Disease Control and the American group psychology did to confuse this is to keep changing the definition! In 1989 and 1990, the CDC published the statistics with old and new definitions separately, so you could quite clearly see how according to the old definition, the incidence of AIDS went up until 1988 and then started coming down. The new definition is a lump added on top. As soon as they noticed people would realize this, they conflated the two definitions. They now give them as if they're the same."

IY: "Why do you think they did this?"

CS: "In order to ensure that people are still sufficiently frightened and that the sacrifice does not stop. We do not want people to understand the dynamics of this illness because that will subvert the sacrifice. Anything that threatens to resolve the situation is fought bitterly as if it is the enemy.

"If you go to a primitive tribe where they are about to sacrifice fourteen babies, and tell them that this will only make them feel good for a day or a week, and then they'll have to sacrifice more, that there are ways to feel better without this sacrifice — you know what they do? They kill you on the spot! Because you are interfering with their sacrificial ritual. Nobody criticizes the sacrificial ritual.

"Every bit of AIDS research that underwrites the group fantasy and continues the sacrifice is approved of."

IY: "Now how do the people participating in the group fantasy know when the fourteen babies have been killed? How do we know when enough is enough?"

CS: "It's really interesting. The only answer we have is based on work done with other cultures. When, during the Aztec Empire, the priests performed their ritual sacrifice — which they did a lot! — they would take the skulls of the victims, make holes in the temples and fix them onto long poles which they would string up in front of the big pyramid in such a way that whoever stood on top of the pyramid could look down as they imagined the gods would, and could count the skulls on a device called a tzompantli. They literally imagined the gods counting the sacrifices. When the people felt sufficient relief from their bad feelings, this would be conveyed to the High Priest who would then go up on the pyramid, commune with the gods, and declare that the gods have said 'Enough!'"

IY: "So this is literally a Golgotha, a hill of skulls."

CS: "Absolutely. And this is what the Quilt is for AIDS. You display the Quilt, horizontally, to the gods so they can see when enough people have been sacrificed and send the message, 'Stop the sacrifice!' This is exactly the same as the tzompantli. *You are displaying the equivalent of the skulls to the gods so they can decide when there are enough.*

"Group fantasies are relayed through indirect means. Now, since the epidemic is clearly diminishing, they have displayed the Quilt in its entirety for the last time — on the week of October 12 (1992)."[2]

Casper Schmidt finished the interview by saying that he had been treating a number of people with AIDS, and had shared his preliminary findings with fellow therapists in a paper entitled "Guidelines for the Psychoanalytic Treatment of AIDS". In this paper, he observed that his AIDS patients had all suffered syndromes of longstanding stress connected with conflicting feelings about their sexuality and that this condition involved "activation of the hypothalamo-pituitary-adrenal axis (the stress axis)", leading to increased cortisol production and decreased DHEAS. From these beginnings, he traced the course of the cellular disturbance that eventually leads to the gradual, relentless decline in T-cells characteristic of AIDS.

---

[2]Newspaper articles published around this time pointed out that the Quilt had become too big to display whole, in a single location. Since then, new locations have been found, most recently Washington, DC — October 1996.

A visitor to the Quilt on 12 October 1996 wrote anonymously in the guest book: "please god let this be the last time we have to come to washington to see the quilt. no more deaths."

All of these patients, Schmidt found, suffered from intense, socially-induced shame, and an extraordinary capacity to disguise and feign feelings, with negative feelings being "shunted into their bodies", resulting in histories of psychosomatic complaints, and a "suicide syndrome" of "destructive affects ... turned against the self". He also observed that all these patients had been severely traumatized in childhood.

Schmidt was hoping that by combining experimental therapeutic work with a thorough program of nutrition and vitamin supplementation (such as the Direct AIDS Alternative Information Resources Protocol), the core AIDS symptom of continuing T-cell decline might be arrested, and even reversed. And he was hopeful that the incoming Clinton administration would effect positive changes.

After I finished the interview and left Casper's apartment, I walked a few blocks to a friend's place. My friend had just returned from visiting someone he knew, another PWA. "Poor Bob", he said, "he has these terrible lesions here." He pressed his fingers against his temples and made circular motions against the sides of his head. I thought immediately of the holes in the temples of Casper's Aztec skulls — a sudden synchronicity that gave me an eerie feeling — puzzling, and strangely exciting — like the first breakthrough in the cracking of a complex and difficult code.

Casper and I found we had a lot in common, including our love of poetry and South Africa (where I had lived as a child), and we soon became friends. We discussed editing and publishing a book of his short stories, to be entitled *The Barbecue of Madame Nhu,* in reference to a comment by the wife of the President of South Vietnam when monks began to immolate themselves in protest against the war: "I hope they invite me to the barbecue!" Another of his stories was a Borgesian fable about the forgotten origins of the tango among homosexual gauchos during the long, cold nights on the pampas!

I arranged for Casper to spend a holiday visiting me and my partner in Banff during the summer; he was to bring his stories with him. He never arrived, and my efforts to reach him were unsuccessful. What he hadn't told me was that at some point in his researches, he realized, to his horror, that he was diagnosing himself.

The last year or so of Casper's life remains something of a mystery. Diagnosed with AIDS, he entered hospital, and shortly afterwards left, to die at home of AIDS-related illness in the late Spring of 1994, about eighteen months after our interview. The long-promised second part to "The Group-Fantasy Origins of AIDS" was never completed. All his research papers, manuscripts and patient case files have disappeared.

CHAPTER VI

Programmed To Die: Cultural Hypnosis & AIDS[1]

By Michael Ellner and Andrew Cort

Most people incorrectly believe that the "Human Immunodeficiency Virus" (HIV) is synonymous with the "Acquired Immune Deficiency Syndrome" (AIDS), and that AIDS always equals death. There is an AIDS Establishment that thrives on fear and misrepresentation in the name of science and truth.

People with AIDS fears are systematically inundated with the worst possible suggestions, some of which are insidiously subtle. As health care professionals we see the deleterious effects of these suggestions. A person's unconscious beliefs powerfully affect that person's response to illness, including AIDS. For example, suppose a person with AIDS (PWA) makes changes in behavior, giving up bad habits and concentrating on health and healing. This could very well improve the PWA's chances for a long and healthy life. But let's say that hidden under the surface is this PWA's belief that it's hopeless, that nothing can be done, that any effort is in vain. These unconscious beliefs could totally undermine the healthy behavior and positive, conscious intentions. This is a working model of self-hypnosis. No trance or hypnotist is needed.

---

[1]This essay was written in 1990, and has been published in several newsletters since then.

Bone-pointing, or voodoo death, is a well documented hypnotic phenomenon that clearly demonstrates the awesome power of belief. There are people in Africa, Haiti, and Australia with the belief that the shaman (or witch doctor) has power over life and death. For them, being the target of a bone pointed by such an authority, can be fatal. The hex is harmless to a non-believer; but to a believer it is deadly. After having a bone pointed at them, healthy people go home and obediently die.

In our culture, doctors and the media have considerable authority, and people usually accept their suggestions, both the overt ones and the subtle ones. We place extraordinary trust in our medical experts and the press. And if they tell us over and over again that "AIDS is always fatal" and nothing can be done, it makes a deep and lasting and lethal impression.

But the facts show that up to 20% of people with full-blown AIDS are continuing to live full and active lives six or more years after diagnosis. AIDS is not, and has never been "always fatal". This titillating, sensationalist assumption is based on inaccurate information.[2]

We are not saying that anyone is intentionally or with conscious malice programming PWAs or HIV-seropositives to die. We are pointing out that it is possible for people to follow the expected course of AIDS simply because they believe what they hear. They give up! This is also an example of cooperation with the accepted cultural authorities and a validation of one's faith in science and our society. Our public health and media policies concerning AIDS are like "electronic bone-pointing". Keep in mind that repetition plays a large role in the hypnotic

---

[2]According to CDC statistics, some people diagnosed with "AIDS" in the first years of the epidemic are still alive now, over a decade later.

process. We all have plenty of unhealthy beliefs that make us vulnerable to a barrage of doom and gloom.

Another abuse is the use of the phrases "AIDS virus" and "AIDS test". No virus (or any other agent) has been proved by science to be the inevitable cause of AIDS. No test now exists which can tell you if you are going to develop the disease. There are many qualified medical experts who do not believe that HIV is solely responsible for the complex syndrome, and some top scientists believe that HIV is not even harmful.[3]

A false impression is being perpetuated, that we understand what causes this disease. But before a particular germ (bacterium, virus or fungus) can be considered the cause of a particular disease, there are certain standards of proof, known as Koch's Postulates, which must be met. The first of Koch's Postulates (which amounts to good common sense) stipulates: "The germ must be found growing abundantly in every patient and every diseased tissue."[4] When the First Postulate cannot be fulfilled, the other postulates are irrelevant, because the germ cannot be the cause of the disease. The HIV-Causes-AIDS hypothesis is also soundly refuted by the evidence of molecular biology: the virus is consistently inactive, even in patients who are dying of AIDS.[5] And finally, the hypothesis that HIV causes AIDS is refuted by epidemiology: AIDS is simply not behaving like an infectious disease; it has never spread from the original "risk groups" into the general population.

---

[3]Especially see the works of Peter Duesberg, listed in Appendix A.

[4]The logic of Koch's First Postulate is explained cogently in Duesberg's book, *Inventing The AIDS Virus,* Washington, DC: Regnery 1996.

[5]See Duesberg, *Inventing The AIDS Virus.*

No one knows what a positive result on the HIV-antibody tests (Elisa and Western Blot) really means. HIV seropositive people, who are now healthy, may just be vaccinated. If they continue to take good care of their health, they may very well be safe from any potential illnesses associated with AIDS, and may live to a ripe old age.[6]

AIDS has become a major industry. Millions of dollars are being made and spent on research and drugs based on an unproven assumption about HIV. It is as if we were, dare we say, hypnotized. Many people have their reputations and livelihoods invested in the HIV theory. These same people control all the research and all the research funds. They are also the people with direct access to the media, so they are in a position to shape our beliefs and expectations.. Healthy asymptomatic people, who merely test positive for an HIV antibody, are being persuaded to take a dangerous and toxic drug, AZT, in hope that it will buy them more time.[7] AZT also happens to be

---

[6]Eleni Papadopulos-Eleopulos, et al., "Is a Western Blot Proof of HIV Infection?", *Bio/Technology*, June 1993, pp. 691-707.

This article provides a devastating critique of the commonly used "HIV-antibody" tests, the Elisa and the Western Blot. Neither of these tests has ever been *validated* against the only meaningful standard, actual isolation of the retrovirus HIV. This means that no one knows exactly what these tests actually measure. Nevertheless, these tests are the basis for an assumption of "HIV infection" and for treatment with highly toxic nucleoside analogue drugs (AZT, ddI, ddC, d4T, etc.) — drugs which are capable of killing the patient, even though he might be perfectly healthy prior to treatment.

[7]See various articles by John Lauritsen, especially Chapter II: "AZT On Trial", in *Poison By Prescription: The AZT Story*, Asklepios 1990; and Chapter XXIX: "FDA Documents Show Fraud In AZT Trials" in *The AIDS War*, Asklepios 1993.

the most expensive drug in the history of medicine. Yet this drug, has never been shown, by rigorous scientific standards, to be effective.

The good news is that once you become aware that you are harboring false and dangerous beliefs about HIV and AIDS, it is possible to change them. You might wish to look into the life-affirming applications of hypnosis and self-hypnosis.[8] You may also wish to experience the benefits of the various complementary healing arts, as well as taking the obvious steps of treating yourself with good nutrition, exercise, avoidance of drugs, and a general life-style of good health habits.

We hope we have given you some food for thought concerning HIV and AIDS. It is quite possible to be programmed to die. It is also possible to be programmed to live. Before closing, we want to say clearly that safer sex and other precautions are a good idea. AIDS is a multifaceted problem requiring a variety of health-affirming responses. We do not want to let the AIDS medical and media establishment scare you to death.

Also see Duesberg, *Inventing The AIDS Virus*, for a clear explanation of how AZT works, biochemically, as a non-selective terminator of DNA synthesis.

[8]You are best served by consulting a certified hypnotherapist. Do not assume that a person with an MD, PhD, MSW or CSW degree is qualified to practise hypnosis.

CHAPTER VII

Deadly Counsels: The Necrophiliacs of "AIDS"[1]

by Cass Mann

On Friday 13th September, as part of the Wellcome-sponsored[2] "Fifth International Conference for People with HIV/-AIDS", a "Celebration of Life" was held at Westminster Abbey. Although the event was promoted as a multi-denominational gathering for an international audience, the service itself was entirely Christian. Only Christian hymns and psalms were featured, thus causing anguish for the many non-Christians present, who realized the utter inappropriateness of the event for themselves. Most chilling of all, and the greatest offence to people living with "HIV" and "AIDS", was the reading from Dr. Elisabeth Kubler-Ross's *AIDS: The Ultimate Challenge*, a work that has become the bible in "AIDS counselling":

> Is it possible that people with HIV and AIDS, children and adults alike, *chose* to contribute their *short* life spans on planet Earth to help us to open our eyes, to raise our consciousness, to open our heart and minds, and finally to see the light? [Emphasis added.]

---

[1]An earlier version of this article was published in *MAINLINERS* (London), November 1991.

[2]That is, Wellcome Pharmaceuticals, the manufacturer of AZT.

No, Kubler Ross. *No!* People with "HIV" and "AIDS" did *not* "choose" to have "HIV" or "AIDS" as an educational tool for humanity, or to be topics of conversation for the new-age dinner party set, as to what these gorgeously pathetic people are contributing to "open our hearts and minds". It is as revolting a proposition as to imagine that the Jews, on their way to the Nazi concentration camps, skipped along singing: *"We're here to teach the world to sing, in perfect harmony."*

I declare that the greatest danger to people living with "HIV" and "AIDS" is the wholesale pollution of "AIDS" counselling by the death-promoting and life-negating philosophy of such counsellors as Kubler-Ross, whose disciples have been placed in practically all the major UK "AIDS" counselling agencies, with tragic consequences. When people come to them for advice, the Kubler-Ross counsellors tell them to prepare for their own imminent death, which, they unscientifically claim, inevitably follows a diagnosis of being HIV-antibody positive.

It is woefully apparent that most "AIDS" counselling agencies and organizations have deliberately chosen to ignore the growing body of evidence that "AIDS" is *not* inevitably fatal, and that individuals with "AIDS" diagnoses can recover and are doing so. Instead, London Lighthouse, the UK's leading "AIDS" counselling and training agency, fully incorporates the Kubler-Ross view when declaring:

> The primary focus of London Lighthouse's work is the empowerment of people affected by HIV and AIDS ... [by working] to change ingrained social attitudes which collude to deny that death and dying are central facets of life and living.

The unstated assumption here is that "death and dying" are the inevitable outcome of an HIV-antibody-positive diagnosis, in full and flagrant ignorance of the evidence that this is *not* the case. Through such an approach, the Lighthouse/Kubler-Ross counsellors endeavor to destroy hope, under a hypocritical posture of combatting *denial* of "death and dying".

Lighthouse's original launch statement was even clearer on this point:

> London Lighthouse's main aim is to offer an integrated range of services to care for people from their *initial* diagnosis of HIV infection through to providing a supportive and loving environment where people can die with dignity. [Emphasis added.]

It is here implied that there is a linear progression, which can be summed up in a formula promoted by most "AIDS" counsellors: HIV = AIDS = DEATH.

Kevin Waite, Lighthouse's Welfare Adviser, writes in *Pink Paper* (23 February 1991):

> Those who are HIV+ and who are *able* and wish to work part-time are, consequently, on low incomes. [Emphasis added.]

The same assumption is made of an inevitable descent into illness following a diagnosis of "HIV+". Note well the expectation that "HIV+" people are able to work only part-time, if at all.

In *Body Positive Newsletter* (*BPN*, 18 June 1991), "The Natural Death Centre" in London was promoted in this way:

> The Centre hopes to break the taboo around death and *encourage* people to prepare for death in workshops, literature, will-creating and a support network. [Emphasis added.]

BPN's Editor-in-Chief Mark Crowther wrote an article on relationships entered into by those who have been diagnosed as "HIV-antibody positive":

> We [people with HIV] have a subconscious fear that we aren't worth loving, and cannot understand how someone could love us in spite of our status. The fact that our condition is potentially fatal makes this all the more real. Who would want to go out with someone who might drop dead? What's the point in starting something when the church service that finalizes the union might be a funeral rather than a wedding? [*BPN*, 26 March 1991]

Fellow *BPN* editor Peter Johnson writes in the same issue:

> HIV begins a decline in the immune system that results in increasingly serious diseases. You can think of it as a slide down a slope from healthy mountain air at the top to a polluted soup at the valley bottom. [*BPN*, 26 March 1991]

When you get to the "polluted soup at the valley bottom", don't neglect to "swirl around in a cesspool of your own making", in the anti-gay words of Police Chief James Anderton, whose outlook on "AIDS" is strikingly similar to that of Johnson's.

In contrast to all of these unscientific, death-promoting statements, the discoverer of HIV, Dr. Luc Montagnier, had this to say:

> AIDS does not inevitably lead to death, especially if you suppress the co-factors that support the disease. It's very important to tell this to people who are infected. Psychological factors are critical in supporting immune function. If you suppress this psychological support by telling someone he is condemned to die, your words alone will have condemned him. It simply isn't true that the virus is one hundred percent fatal. [*Positively Healthy News*, Issue 2, March 1989]

The "ingrained social attitudes", alluded to earlier, do not collude to *deny* death and dying; they unashamedly *promote* them. Sixty million people worldwide were recently glued to their television sets, gloating over a blatant promotion of death and dying; they were "colluding" in the potential death or serious injury of one or two boxers. Many of the same people would have torn limb-from-limb the same two boxers if, instead of attempting to murder each other in the ring, they had made love to each other. The love of death and hatred of life sells newspapers and creates bestsellers; Rambo becomes a cult-hero, while the victims of violence become martyrs and saints.

Death and dying are favored issues with "AIDS" counsellors, presenting facile, non-political solutions to the troublesome practical and emotional problems people living with "HIV" and "AIDS" diagnoses face. The Kubler-Ross clones choose to ignore the philosophy of self-empowerment, exemplified by the "AIDS-activist" movement, since this goes counter to their touted acceptance of death and dying. By harping on death and dying, the counsellors focus the counselling discourse in areas that will not expose their own ignorance. By spouting platitudes, they avoid the necessity of researching the enormous body of data pertaining to "AIDS".

How many of the deaths, especially the suicides, of people with "HIV" or "AIDS", have been caused by the deadly psychopathology underlying most "AIDS" counselling? It is a terrible thing psychologically to present someone with the expectation that, from the moment of his "HIV-positive" diagnosis, he is one of the living dead, awaiting only the formalities of cremation and memorial service. Shamefully, most "AIDS" organizations go along with this fabrication as — in order to be acceptable to the bodies that fund them — they have made pacts to accept the prevailing "AIDS" dogmas, and to expunge heretical and activist elements from their midst.

Surviving, Getting Better, Staying Healthy

Up to this point I have been describing a mind-set among those involved in "AIDS" counselling, for whose end product I shall coin the diagnosis: *Death By Counselling.*

Is there an antidote to this poisonous counselling? There is, and it consists of re-programming along the following lines:

1. *Don't accept that having "HIV" or "AIDS" is a death sentence.*

Robert Gallo, the other co-discoverer of HIV, has gone on record as stating that 67% of forms of HIV are not pathogenic and will not cause disease in the lifetime of the host. Why, then, are we all assuming that the form of HIV we were diagnosed with is *the* pathogenic form? Because we were programmed to do so by certain doctors, counsellors and organizations.

A rapidly growing number of scientists, writers and others — belonging to the Rethinking AIDS group based in California — have come to reject the HIV-causes-AIDS hypothesis. Some of them believe that HIV is not harmful at all.

2. Question the medical knowledge and scientific accuracy of all "AIDS" data you have been presented with.

There is much disagreement regarding "AIDS", its causes and treatments. Even the ultra-conservative *Sunday Telegraph* admitted in an article, "Fears rise that HIV treatments hasten death", that the prevailing "AIDS" model is beginning to crumble:

> Evidence is mounting that scientists have misunderstood the way the Aids virus [*sic*] attacks humans, raising fears that some treatments now being developed may actually hasten death ... The conventional view of Aids ... has run into trouble.... Since the earliest days of Aids research, there have been some puzzling features of the disease.... Scientists have been misled.... Criticism of the MRC's [Medical Research Council] Aids programme is growing. (*Sunday Telegraph*, 22 September 1991)

You should be aware that some of the leading "AIDS experts" have been found guilty of "scientific misconduct" or fraud, or have been convicted or placed under indictment for felonies. You should be aware further that most "AIDS" research has been of poor quality, and in some cases fraudulent.

There does not exist even a single study that clearly and unambiguously demonstrates benefits for any of the nucleoside analogues (AZT, ddI, ddC, d4T, d3T, etc.). Virtually all of the studies which claim to show *slight* benefits for these drugs were paid for and controlled by their manufacturers.

3. Find out what people living healthily with HIV/AIDS are doing with their lives.

There are many more of them than you have been allowed to know existed: people who overcame their diagnoses of "AIDS" or "HIV-antibody-positive" — who have recovered their health and are staying healthy. They are fighters, tough and streetwise, who will not allow themselves to be used as experimental laboratory animals for the testing of toxic drugs for multinational pharmaceutical companies. They have absolutely no truck with the death-dealing "AIDS" culture.

These long-term survivors have been vividly and excellently described by "AIDS" activist and singer/songwriter Michael Callen, who has lived with "AIDS" for over ten years, in his book, *Surviving AIDS* (New York 1990). The one characteristic he found common to all the survivors he interviewed was *grit:*

> These people were all fighters: skeptical, opinionated, incredibly knowledgeable about AIDS, and passionately committed to living. They have worked hard to stay alive. They were all pragmatic optimists; they frequently reported that they had what is commonly referred to as "the right attitude", which basically meant that they had hope.

Callen's survivors were cautious and skeptical about medical drugs. Only one of them had ever tried AZT (except very briefly, abandoning it at the first sign of toxicity) — "despite unbelievably intense pressure to do so". They also (with only two exceptions) "profoundly curtailed their use of recreational drugs and alcohol soon after diagnosis".

Sadly, four of Callen's approximately 30 survivors died between the time he did his interviews and the time his book was finished. Three of them had been persuaded by peer pressure to go on AZT; the fourth had continued to take drugs and drink heavily.

Callen discusses the new discipline, initiated by Dr. George Solomon in 1964, of Psycho-neuroimmunology (PNI), the science of the relationship of mind and body — which proposes that thoughts and emotions profoundly affect the course of a disease by strengthening or weakening the complex immune responses of the body. More simply stated: *Attitudes affect outcome.*

As a result of one-to-one work with over five hundred people with "HIV-antibody-positive" or "AIDS" diagnoses, I can say — very simply — that in order to live healthily with "HIV / AIDS":

> ***Only have in your life that which supports and celebrates your aims and purposes, and detach immediately from everything which doesn't.***

Necrophilia versus Biophilia

The following is taken from Matthew Fox's fascinating book, *Original Blessing,* a treatise on "creation-centered spirituality":

> What has been most lacking in society and religion in the West for the past six centuries has been a *Via Positiva,* a way or path of affirmation, thanksgiving, ecstasy. These are more than conceptual themes, however. They are journeys, deeply entered into, deeply felt, and deeply shareable. They are

> journeys of life, not death; of awareness, not numbness; of Eros, not control. And therefore they are journeys of ... healing power. The Via Positiva is a way of tasting the beauties and cosmic depths of creation, meaning ourselves and everything else. Without this solid grounding in creation's powers we become bored, violent people. We become necrophiliacs in love with death and the powers and principalities of death.

In a culture which prefers necrophilia (love of death) to biophilia (love of life), it is no surprise that the first response to the "AIDS epidemic" was to teach people with "HIV"/"AIDS" *how to die well*; what it was actually doing was teaching them how to *die while well*. People who may never have been acknowledged for anything else in their lifetimes were suddenly being feted for their unique ability to "die well". Books such as Allegra Taylor's *Acquainted With The Night* were written to celebrate their ignorance regarding alternative reality-models to "dying well". This pollution reached even the "alternative medicine" press, as in the Summer 1991 issue of *Caduceus* — an issue dedicated to necrophilia — we find an article on London's "communities for the dying", which featured London Lighthouse, The Christian Community and Mildmay Mission Hospice. Interestingly, Mildmay's Rev. Peter Clarke stated: *"Some patients may come in medically in a bit of a mess."*

The concept of preventing the patient from being in such a state in the first place is sadly beyond the comprehension of most "AIDS" counsellors. However, the most revealing interview was with Khaldun Nahr of Lighthouse, "who heads a team of four full-time counsellors". In his own words:

"There was one man who had AIDS and was dying. He had stunning eyes; just like stars. They sparkled and shone. I'd never seen anyone with eyes like that. He was sick of being sick. He was fed up with the pain and suffering and exhaustion and wanted to die. Everything he said made sense — I couldn't find a reason to tell him to fight on. Intuitively I said, 'I see you as the man with incredible eyes. And because they're still sparkling and shining, it just makes me wonder if you have something left to see.'" Nahr added, "No one cares that I've got a PhD. People care only that we care about them. Knowing that, they feel safe in professional hands."

Oh yeah? Think again, mister! No one gives a damn about your PhD or flourishes of poetry. Where is the evidence of earlier intervention by "AIDS" counsellors in Mr. Sparkling Eyes' treatment protocol? What about the possibility that his wanting to die may have been the tragic outcome of toxic treatments prescribed by his medical practitioners, worsened by fatal nutritional advice by dietitians and nutritionists? While great professional support is available to those wanting to die, the concept of preventing people from being so devastated in the first place — medically and psychologically — seems to be beyond the experience of those in the "AIDS" counselling profession.

For all those who have condemned us to die, the following message: LIVING IS THE BEST REVENGE!

Afterword (August 1996):

Re-reading this article five years later I am struck with how little the HIV=AIDS=DEATH model has changed and how little progress has been made in uncovering the mysteries of how HIV could cause AIDS all by itself. Nevertheless, on scientifically untenable grounds, the AIDS counselling profession continues to insist that the most appropriate response to an HIV antibody-positive diagnosis is to prepare for one's own death.

The only change is that a longer time span between diagnosis and death is now allowed, since many more HIV Positives than expected are stubbornly refusing to die on cue.

It may be interesting to update the reader as to what became of the people mentioned in the article. Kubler Ross has, to all intents and purposes, burnt out and retired from the fray after her ranch was burnt down, but she still remains the biggest, and most pernicious, influence in AIDS counselling. Khaldun Nahr PhD has resigned from London Lighthouse, as has its founder, Christopher Spence. Both Mark Crowther and Peter Johnson of Body Positive have died.

Those who survive and thrive after their diagnoses have had hard lessons to learn, of which the most difficult to accept is this: *Being a gay man today in a commercial gay culture is in and of itself a toxic and dangerous condition.* The trivialization and infantilization of gay men — their reduction to fetishistic body-fascist sex objects clamoring to put on the chains successfully cast off by the revolutionary women's liberation movement — makes living after 40 an undesirable state of affairs. Add to this mix an allegedly fatal virus, which makes aging unnecessary (there is no concept in gay culture of maturity), and you have the perfect exit line. As writer Edmund White observes, "There are no gay men over 40 in New York". And very few gay men over 40 anywhere else that "queer culture" has established itself, who truly, madly, deeply want to live beyond this age. The saddest lesson we have learnt is that the greatest danger to gay men is not HIV, but the way gay men prey on and demean one another. In this context, AIDS is not the worst thing that could happen.

CHAPTER VIII

HIV Voodoo From Burroughs Wellcome[1]

John Lauritsen

Those who have eyes to see are witnessing genocide — the genocide of gay men. Millions of dollars are now being spent on an international advertising campaign, "Living With HIV", in which gay men and other members of "risk groups" are being told: Get tested for antibodies to HIV — if you "test positive" you need "medical intervention", which could "put time on your side". The "medical intervention" is AZT (also known as Retrovir and zidovudine), and the campaign is paid for, directly and indirectly, by Burroughs-Wellcome, the manufacturer of AZT.[2]

The campaign consists of a phoney diagnosis followed by a lethal treatment. Already tens of thousands of objectively healthy gay men have been scared and bullied and bamboozled into taking AZT, allegedly in order to "slow the progression to

---

[1]This article was originally published in the *New York Native,* 7 January 1991, and was reprinted as Chapter XXIII of *The AIDS War.*

[2]Developed as cancer chemotherapy in the 60s, AZT was designed to kill all growing cells through the termination of DNA synthesis (described excellently in Peter Duesberg's *Inventing The AIDS Virus*, Appendix A). Normally chemotherapy is given for only a few days or weeks. The hope is that the drugs will kill the cancerous cells in the patient's body before killing the patient himself — and that, after the drugs have been stopped, the patient will be able to recover from the poisoning without the cancer. However, in the case of AZT therapy for "AIDS", the poison is administered for as long as the patient lives.

AIDS". Optimism regarding their prognosis would be foolish. Except for the lucky few who stop "treatment" in time, they will die. Death is the inevitable biochemical consequence of taking AZT, for the fundamental action of the drug is to terminate DNA synthesis, the very life process itself. Without a single benefit demonstrated by honest and competent research, AZT can do nothing but kill.

It is odd, the power of words to cloud reality or discredit a line of reasoning. A British journalist once told me that no one would ever believe what I wrote if I persisted in using words like "genocide". My response is that I write what I consider to be true, not necessarily what will be believable. Genocide has occurred at other times and in other places, and it is happening here and now, whether or not people wish to believe it.

Craig Schoonmaker, the founder of Homosexuals Intransigent, has suggested the word "autogenocide", to emphasize the role of low self-esteem and self-hatred in motivating gay men to acquiesce in their own destruction. Casper Schmidt, a New York City psychiatrist, has proposed "pharmacogenocide": genocide through drugs. The late Robert Mendelsohn put forward the word "iatrogenocide" in his best seller, *Confessions of a Medical Heretic*:

> A new word was recently coined by Dr. Quentin Young to describe one activity of Modern Medicine: iatrogenocide. Iatrogenocide (*iatros* is the Greek for doctors) is the systematic destruction of a large group of people by doctors.[3]

[3]Robert S. Mendelsohn, *Confessions of a Medical Heretic*, Chicago 1979.

This new form of genocide, directed against gay men, rests on two pillars: Homophobia and Profit. The ancient taboo from the *Holiness Code of Leviticus*, which prescribed the death penalty for males who had sex with each other, is now being carried out, profitably, by the pharmaceutical industry:

> "If a man lie with mankind as with a woman, both of them have committed an abomination: they shall surely be put to death; their blood shall be upon them." (*Leviticus 20:13*)

Jewish priests 2500 years ago ordained death by stoning for the "abomination" of sex between males. Modern priests, the doctors, prescribe AZT, with the extraordinarily hypocritical dogma that by giving a life-terminating drug they are really "extending life". Considering the agonizing side effects of AZT "treatment", it might be argued that death by stoning were preferable.

Deadly diagnosis + lethal treatment = genocide

Behind the scenes a growing number of important scientists are now convinced that HIV is not the cause of "AIDS". The two "discoverers" of HIV, Luc Montagnier of the Pasteur Institute and Robert Gallo on the National Cancer Institute, have both reneged on promises to defend the HIV-AIDS hypothesis against the criticisms of Peter Duesberg.[4]

What does it mean to be diagnosed as "HIV positive"? Objectively it means nothing more than *possibly* having antibodies to

---

[4]See Appendix A.

a harmless passenger virus. In the absence of "medical treatment" or other specific health risks, there is no reason why someone who is "HIV positive" should not live to a ripe old age.[5]

The "HIV positive" diagnosis itself, however, can be deadly. It has led to suicides, has destroyed marriages and careers, and is used to justify AZT treatment. An East Berlin writer recently summed it up with the phrase, *"Nicht das Virus, sondern die Diagnose tötet"*. ("The virus doesn't kill, the diagnosis does.")[6]

The acute (short-term) toxicities of AZT are serious, and many patients die of them. These toxicities include severe anemia, muscle disease, and damage to the kidneys, liver, and nerves. However, it is the chronic (long-term) toxicities that are of most concern when AZT is being prescribed for healthy people to take for the rest of their lives. The cumulative, long-term effects of

---

[5]The "HIV-antibody" tests, Elisa and Western Blot, have never been *validated* against the only meaningful standard, actual isolation of the virus itself. (Tests themselves are supposed to be tested before they are put into use. "Validation" in this context is a technical term: To validate a test means to answer the question, "What exactly does this test measure?") In fact, the alleged "HIV-antibody" tests cross-react with many different antigens formed in the body, which have nothing whatever to do with HIV. Someone who has been vaccinated for the flu, or has ever had malaria or leprosy, or has a history of substance abuse, may very well score positive on the Elisa and/or the Western Blot. In addition, the tests are highly unreliable, even for measuring whatever it is that they do measure. (See Papadopulos-Eleopulos *et al.*, Appendix A.)

[6]Erhard Neubert, *"Kunstprodukt 'AIDS' in Schwierigkeiten"* ("The Phoney AIDS Construct in Trouble"), *Raum & Zeit* (Space & Time), Special 4, Sauerlach, Germany, October 1990, pages 98-102. (The entire 115-page special issue of *Raum & Zeit* is devoted to German, Swiss, and American AIDS dissidents, who attack the AIDS orthodoxies with much intelligence and militancy. My favorite phrase: *"Nur tote Fische schwimmen mit dem Strom!"* ["Only dead fish swim with the stream!"])

AZT are unknown, since no one has lived for more than three years on AZT treatment. However, the evidence we have — including biochemical analyses, test tube studies, rodent studies, and correlations between cancer of the lymph system and AZT therapy — strongly indicates that AZT will cause cancer in the long run.[7]

So then, perfectly healthy members of a group, which is hated for theological reasons, are being persuaded through lies to take a drug that will kill them. If there's a better word than "genocide" to describe this, what is it?

The marketing of genocide

Burroughs-Wellcome's full-page "Living With HIV" advertisements have appeared in *The New York Times* and in lesser publications all over the world. They are found in New York City subways and bus shelters. In a typical ad, a man is shown in silhouette by a grand piano, his head bowed in dejection, and above his head the statement, "I learned I was HIV positive 5 years ago. I felt angry, deserted, and victimized." At the bottom of the ad is an insert photograph of the same man, now smiling and confident: "Today I'm back in control." The theme of "control" is echoed in the ad slogan, "The sooner you take control the better." In all of the "Living With HIV" ads, the body copy is the same:

---

[7]In 1996 it is no longer true that no one has survived longer than three years on AZT. Out of the many tens of thousands of people who have been prescribed AZT, a few have survived longer than this on low doses. However, the generalization remains valid: AZT therapy is incompatible with recovery from "AIDS". There are no reliable, actuarial statistics on survival among those on AZT therapy.

> Every day, more and more people are learning to live with HIV. People are finding ways to stay healthier, strengthen their immune systems, develop positive attitudes. They've found that proper diet, moderate exercise, even stress management can help. And now, early medical intervention could put time on your side.
>
> Today, HIV positive doesn't mean you have to give up. So, the sooner you take control, the better.
>
> For more information on living with HIV, we urge you to call the number below ... anonymously, if you wish.

Such phrases as "stay healthier" and "put time on your side" are insidious, as they suggest that someone with HIV antibodies is already sick and doomed. The references to diet, exercise, and so on are merely window dressing. Any HIV positive who calls the number will find out soon enough that "taking control" means "early medical intervention" means AZT.

In their nauseating hypocrisy, the Burroughs-Wellcome ads are reminiscent of a series of ads which in 1983 were run in gay publications for Great Lakes Products, the world's largest manufacturer of poppers (nitrite inhalants). Entitled "Blueprint for Health", the Great Lakes ads gave advice to gay men on how to stay healthy through exercise, nutrition, stress reduction, and so on. And this "message of good health and wellness" was sponsored by the manufacturer of poppers, a drug which, among other things, damages chromosomes; causes anemia, immune suppression, and cardio-vascular collapse; and forms carcinogenic compounds in the body.[8]

---

[8]See Appendix B.

Concomitant with the Burroughs-Wellcome ads, the New York City Department of Health put up posters with the theme, "Living Longer, Staying Strong", conveying essentially the same message, that "people with HIV" are sick and doomed, but might "stay healthy longer" with the help of "early health care and new medicines".

Genocide doesn't take holidays. On Christmas day I was listening to WINS radio, and heard a "Message on HIV" from the Centers for Disease Control (CDC). It was a virtual clone of the "Living with HIV" series. I called the number, and the woman who answered gave me the now-familiar pitch about the importance of getting tested, early medical intervention, and the rest of it.

The gay press promotes autogenocide

Gay publications all over the world, from local bar rags to those with international circulations, are now carrying the "Living with HIV" ads. The *New York Native* and the west coast magazine *Outlook* are the only exceptions I know of. According to an article by Chris Bull in *The Advocate*, Burroughs-Wellcome marketing representative Joe DiSabato found "little opposition to the ads from the gay press." DiSabato richly deserves the 1990 gay Pollyanna prize for his statement, "In a way Burroughs Wellcome is giving money back to the community through the campaign. Economically, this will be great for the gay press."[9]

The German magazine *Magnus* received 20,000 DM to run a Burroughs-Wellcome ad, and a prominent gay activist with

---

[9]DiSabato has since died of an acute asthma attack.

"AIDS" was recruited to assist in the campaign. A Burroughs-Wellcome ad appeared in the latest issue of *Babilonia* (Milan).

In Houston, the Body Positive group received $85,000 plus donations of computers and other equipment from Burroughs-Wellcome. In return, Body Positive ran under its own name a series of television, radio, billboard, and press advertisements with the theme, "We can't get results until you do." For those who would test positive, the ads offered the bleak hope, "There's a chance for a longer and healthier life with early medical intervention." Houston's mayor, Kathy Whitmire, proclaimed September the "Get Tested Now" month, stating that, "prompt medical and psychological intervention can slow down the progress of the [HIV] disease and ameliorate some of its effects."

Some of the ads in the gay press were sponsored by branches of the Public Health Service, paid for with our tax money. One such ad, which ran in *Au Courant* (Philadelphia), contained the following copy:

> Today, people with HIV are doing something most of us didn't think possible. Living longer. Today, a person who is infected with HIV and receives prompt treatment can live longer. If you are at risk [read: if you are gay], now's the time to seek counseling and testing. If you are infected with HIV, work with a doctor to understand medical options that may prolong your life.

The psychology of genocide

In formulating hypotheses on what might be the real causes of "AIDS", multifactorialists who reject the HIV-AIDS hypothesis have concentrated on such probable etiological factors as "recreational" drug use, known and yet-to-be-identified infectious agents, and excessive medical treatment with antibiotics and other drugs. We have, regrettably, tended to slight psychological factors. This is unfortunate, as the concept of psychosomatic illness is well established. There can be no doubt that extreme fear, depression, stress, and grief are capable of causing illness and death.

In 1984 the *Journal of Psychohistory* published a paper by Casper Schmidt, which was perhaps the first to challenge the "AIDS virus" hypothesis.[10] Entitled "The Group-Fantasy Origins of AIDS", this brilliantly original essay advances the thesis that epidemic AIDS has a psychosocial origin — that AIDS is psychologically contagious, being spread through suggestion rather than through microbes. In Schmidt's view, we are witnessing a mass sacrificial ritual, with sadistic persecutors on one side and willing (masochistic) sacrificial victims on the other. The extraordinary irrationality that characterizes the AIDS epidemic can be explained through the concept of group fantasy: people are collectively in a trance.

Schmidt is somewhat more tentative in trying to explain why gay men and other members of "risk groups" are getting sick in ways that qualify for a diagnosis of "AIDS". He proposes that chronic and inescapable fear can elicit a biochemical reaction in the body, which in time causes "psychogenically-reduced cell-mediated immunity". He maintains that this hypothesis has fulfilled the animal model for "AIDS", inasmuch as laboratory animals subjected to inescapable threats have developed immune deficiency. While I withhold judgment on this aspect of Schmidt's

---

[10]Reprinted as Chapter I of this book.

thesis, I wholeheartedly agree that a sacrificial ritual is taking place. Especially noteworthy, in my opinion, is the role of the *facilitators*: those gay men (and lesbians) who are leading the victims to the sacrificial altar, without necessarily allowing themselves to be sacrificed.

In this second wave of sacrifices, in which perfectly healthy people are being targeted for genocide, a crucial role is played by psychological suggestion. Highly sophisticated psychological techniques are being used to make gay men perceive themselves as sick, and become sick, in order to qualify as consumers of AZT. The "Living With HIV" campaign is, quite literally, a form of voodoo.

Michael Ellner, the president of the Health Education AIDS Liaison (HEAL), recently posed the question of whether unrecognized hypnosis might not be a risk factor in the development of "AIDS". A certified master hypnotherapist himself, Ellner believes that classic elements of hypnosis are present in the "Living With HIV" campaign, in innumerable pronouncements from AIDS groups and public health agencies, and in a recent video from Burroughs-Wellcome (about which more below). Ellner cited the elements of hypnotism as being, in no particular order: perceived authority, fixation, suggestion, repetition, confusion, relaxation, imagination, and post-hypnotic suggestion.

A Burroughs-Wellcome video: Brainwashing the doctors

A few months ago, doctors who treat AIDS patients received a video cassette from Burroughs-Wellcome, "The Psychology of Treating Patients With HIV Disease". The basic premises of the video are the same as those of the "Living With HIV" campaign, that "HIV infection" and "AIDS" are more or less equivalent, and that early medical intervention (with AZT / Retrovir) is called for. Beyond this, doctors are told to "ally with the treatment", by knocking down any hesitation or objections their "HIV-infected" patients might have to going and staying on AZT therapy.

The video is narrated by Leon McKusick, Ph.D., a gay psychologist in San Francisco. His voice is heard saying:

> HIV disease is coming to be seen as a chronic infection. And for many individuals this is the first intimate realization of death and disease, particularly among those who are relatively young.

After McKusick introduces himself, he quickly gets to the point:

> The decisions surrounding the initiation of Retrovir therapy force you, the physician, to evaluate the patient's support network.... This video will share with you the psychological reactions we've seen from patients who are diagnosed positive for the HIV antibodies, and then alert you to the emotions that follow as they encounter the progression of the disease and then are motivated towards treatment with Retrovir.

McKusick describes "HIV-related depression", emphasizing that the symptoms mimic those of HIV infection itself, as well as "some of the early side effects of AZT". In other words, if a patient on AZT should experience sleep disturbance, eating problems, fatigue, or weight loss, these might be merely short-term "HIV-related depression", rather than side effects of AZT.

For physicians to "assist individuals going through emotional depression reacting to HIV or going on treatment", McKusick offers the following guidelines: enlightened reassurance, cognitive reframing, social support, reinforce structure, plan of action. In commenting on the video, Michael Ellner has expressed the opinion that "cognitive reframing" means hypnotizing or brainwashing the patient.

The video features a panel discussion, with two doctors and a number of people with AIDS (PWAs). Like McKusick, the other two authority figures are gay and are identified with title: Marcus Conant, M.D., and Ron Grossman, M.D., whereas the PWAs are identified simply as "Bob", "Steve", "Tom", and "Bill". Drs. McKusick, Conant and Grossman are understanding facilitators. Bob, Steve, Tom, and Bill are willing victims.

Grossman argues that "AIDS" ought to be renamed as "HIV spectrum". His colleagues nod solemnly.

McKusick says, "Sometimes it's best to combat feelings of stigmatization with a sense of humor." He smiles. The camera shifts to Conant, who tries to smile, but his face is heavy and his eyes are dead tired. And then Bob tells an anecdote. It seems he was in a play-writing workshop when the timer of his AZT pill box went off:

> Twenty pairs of eyes zeroed in on me. The only thing I could do, I took out the pill box and turned it off — and they were still looking — so obviously I had to respond to it — so I made a joke out of it. I said, "It's a phenomenon of the latter part of the 20th century in the United States. Every four hours, gay men start to beep."

Bob stops speaking. It becomes apparent that the point of his joke has been made, and that people are expected to laugh. They begin laughing. The camera goes from one person to another to show them laughing. They applaud Bob's performance.

Clearly Bob is intended to be a role model. He states, "As soon as I started taking action, I started feeling better.... Action is the key to salvation."

The prickly topic of AZT's side effects is raised. McKusick asserts that the physician's role ought to be "helping the patient realize that their [*sic*] fears were unfounded." Bob makes a joke about "horror stories" of side effects. Everyone laughs.

McKusick then declares that anxiety symptoms are very much like both HIV symptoms and early symptoms of AZT side effects. He artfully sows confusion by stating:

> Sometimes a person could benefit medically from the drug, but could reject the drug for psychological reasons. Some patients, who have just begun AZT, have complained about side effects which, once they've talked about it with their counsellors, were determined to be more related to their anxiety about being on the drug, than to the drug itself.... Sometimes a person could benefit medically from the treatment, but rejects the drug for psychological reasons, after being on it for just a brief period. Therefore, it's important to recognize that some of your patients' early reactions may be psychological.

Bob makes his contribution: "I have to say — Thank God! — that I have had no side effects whatsoever." Bob is not well. His skin is stretched taut over a death's head, and his facial expressiveness is limited to rolling his eyes. He mentions a few symptoms, which he attributes to HIV, and says, "I can handle that". He laughs bravely.

McKusick commends Bob on the way he "handles attribution". "It's very important", says McKusick, "to ally with the drug against the disease."

The single most stomach-turning episode in the video is provided by the New York physician, Ron Grossman, who smiles as he delivers the following little speech:

> That pill should be an absolute symbol of life, and not a symbol of "Oh, I've got this...." (Marcus Conant nods in agreement) The whole issue of empowerment here, of people taking charge of their own lives, is involved with this decision making, to take this drug.

To summarize: The whole thrust of the video is to downplay AZT's side effects. Doctors are to dismiss their patients' objections to AZT therapy as "psychological", as short-term depression or anxiety. The loyalty of the doctor should be to Retrovir ("the treatment") rather than to the patient ("the disease"). The hidden message to doctors is that they should not hesitate to kill their patients.

The hidden message to gay men is this: "You are doomed. Be brave, willing sacrificial victims. People will applaud you, and laugh at your jokes. Do not listen to the messages of your body."

Who is responsible?

Unscrupulous pharmaceutical companies, corrupt government officials, venal physicians, stupid and cowardly media people, incompetent and dishonest researchers — none of these things are new. They are business as usual. Where, then, does the buck stop? Who is responsible for pharmacogenocide?

My thinking on this question was altered recently when I read *Confessions of a Medical Heretic* by Robert Mendelsohn, who uncompromisingly places the blame on the members of his own profession:

> Despite the obvious corruption of the drug company/doctor marketing connection, I don't blame the drug companies, the detail men, the government agencies which are supposed to police these activities, or the patients who badger their doctors for drugs. Doctors have enough facts in their possession to know what's going on. Even where the drug is fully tested and the side effects and limitations of the drug are well known, most of the harm is done by doctors indiscriminately prescribing the drug. Doctors, after all, are the ones who claim the sacred power and the ethical superiority that goes with it. The drug companies are in business to make money, and they do that by selling as much of their product as they can at as high a price as they can. And although the drug companies subvert the scientific process through which drugs are tested, certified, and made available to doctors, once the drugs are available, they do let doctors know — albeit subtly — just what these drugs can and cannot do.

All of us who know the truth about AZT will have to do what we can. Friends who are on AZT must be told directly and forcefully that they must get off the drug if they want to live. Public health officials, representatives of AIDS organizations, and various and sundry other "AIDS experts" must be confronted with their lies. Above all, doctors must be persuaded, by whatever means are appropriate, that they have no right to kill their patients with AZT. The buck stops with the AZT-pushing doctors. *They* are responsible.

* * *

Postscript, October 1993: Leon McKusick recently died of "AIDS". He may have believed his own propaganda and taken his own medicine.

CHAPTER IX

Long-Term Survival[1]

Michael Callen

I want to make one thing clear when I talk about long-term survivors: I'm not a scientist. I do not claim that what I will say is "scientific". You might think of me as the Monet of AIDS: I will give you impressions. I think they are worth something, but for you blue-suited people who want to see the data, all I have to offer is what I learned from speaking to actual long-term survivors. Basically, I asked them to tell me, in their own words, why they thought they had survived. Our interviews covered a broad range of possible reasons, and some patterns emerged.

Long-term survivors: the first thing to say is that we exist, though you might not know it if you relied for your information on mainstream media. According to the US government statistics — which you can believe or not; they are not very well kept, but they are all we have — 9% of people with full-blown AIDS live 3 years or more, and 5% live 5 years or more. Unfortunately, there have not been significant improvements in median survival

---

[1]The following was abstracted from a transcript of a talk Michael Callen gave at the international symposium, "AIDS; A Different View" (Amsterdam, May 1992). During that talk Callen held up a plastic sandwich bag filled with capsules, and said he took 56 pills every day. He disclosed that he had recently been diagnosed with Kaposi's sarcoma (KS) of the lungs, and did not expect to live much longer. As it turned out, he survived for another year and a half, dying on 27 December 1993, a dozen years after his initial diagnosis of "AIDS".

since I was diagnosed in 1982. The life expectancy of a person with AIDS has only been extended by 6 months. I personally believe that this 6 months is attributable to our ability to prevent pneumocystis carinii pneumonia, the number one killer of people with AIDS.

The most important thing I learned about long-term survivors is that there definitely is a survivor personality. But I also found exceptions. And that actually made me happy, because it says to me that there is no single way, no recipe, no magic way to become a long-term survivor. I personally believe that each person's AIDS is unique. Each of us probably arrived at it in a slightly different way. We are each biochemically, biologically, genetically unique. And so I never expected that any one approach would work for everybody with AIDS. But the patterns that emerged were fascinating, and I shall describe them to you.

If I had to summarize in one word the common characteristic among survivors, it would be *grit*: these people are incredibly feisty, incredibly knowledgeable, very aggressively involved in the struggle to survive.

They spoke very passionately of what they referred to as "healing partnerships with their health-care providers", by which they meant that they respected the opinions and expertise of the various health-care providers they'd sought out, but they did *not* do something simply because they were told to. In every instance, they wanted to know what their options were and what the possible side-effects were. They had worked out relationships with their health-care providers that permitted a dialogue to go back and forth. And in fact, when you have AIDS, your relationship with your doctor is probably the most important relationship that you have, with the possible exception of your lover. And it is a lot like having a lover: it involves fighting, and being honest about your emotions, and talking. And the long-term survivors that I interviewed were very eloquent about how they had worked over the years to achieve really open and wonderful relationships with their health-care providers.

Every long-term survivor mentioned the phrase "major life-style changes". That meant the obvious: it meant that they immediately started practising safe-sex, to avoid exposure to other possible co-infectious factors. Most of them gave up drugs and alcohol, although some of them not entirely.

Also, among lifestyle changes: a lot of people had dabbled with diet changes, but in almost no instance had anyone been able to persist in a radical diet change.

Everybody talked about, among lifestyle changes, what they called "emotional house cleaning", usually after they had survived their first major opportunistic infection. It represented a crisis to them, and they did some soul searching. They went through their relationships and they either repaired them or ended them. They spoke generally about needing to get rid of people in their lives who refused to support them in their belief that they could survive well beyond statistical projections.

I don't know whether it's true here, but in America Elizabeth Kubler-Ross is very popular, and everybody is an instant expert on dying. There are supposed to be five stages, and people will constantly treat you as if you are in one of the stages, usually denial. If you talk about maybe sticking around longer than the 18 months allotted to you, people will look at you oddly and say, "Yeah, sure!". But long-term survivors were militant about it: they simply wouldn't put up with this negativism. They spoke very movingly about needing to surround themselves with people who would support them in their hope.

Interestingly, another thing that everyone mentioned was that knowledge of another long-term survivor was crucial to maintaining their own belief in long-term survival. And that's really not so mysterious, when you stop to think about it. If you set out to do something that *no* human has ever done, it's a different experience than if you set out to do something that *few* humans have done. *You know that it can be done.*

The most surprising finding among my sample of long-term survivors was a clear rebirth of spirituality. With two exceptions — me and one other guy — all the long-term survivors talked about taking great comfort from their spiritual beliefs. It split almost in half: half had actually returned to the religions of their childhood, although none in a fundamentalist, judgmental way; and the other half spoke more generally of the sense that there was a meaning to suffering, a life after death. And there was no question that they took great comfort from those beliefs.

The long-term survivors were all passionately committed to life. That may sound pretty obvious, but for those of you who may have been around people with AIDS, this is going to sound simplistic, but I can't think of any other way to put it. When a catastrophic illness lands in your lap, you really have two choices: it's either a challenge to live, or challenge to begin dying, and I have seen people make each of these choices. I have seen people give up and die on cue, and I have seen people fight.

I want to be really clear here: there is, among people with AIDS, a shorthand notion, that if you want to be in the long--term survivor sweepstakes, you have to have the right attitude. But nobody ever really defines what that means. What is the right attitude? What I concluded from interviewing four dozen long-term survivors, as friends, is that you do have to have the right attitude: you have to believe in the possibility of survival, and you have to be hopeful and surround yourself with people who love and will support you. That will not, however, guarantee that you are a long-term survivor. The inverse seems to be true, however: I have not yet met a single person, who became a long-term survivor, who did not believe that it was possible.

It was interesting to me that the profile of extraordinary survivors with AIDS was pretty identical to the profile of extraordinary survivors of other so-called terminal diseases.

About half of the long-term survivors were in long-term loving relationships, and those who were spoke about how they could not envision going through AIDS alone. They took tremendous comfort and support from their loved ones — practical as well as emotional support.

All of the long-term survivors had dabbled with non-allopathic medicine. Most of them integrated allopathic and non-allopathic medicine. Out of the 48 people I interviewed intensively, only one survivor had completely turned his back on Western medicine and refused to take any pharmaceutical. And I have to say that he is still alive and glows with health. He is probably the healthiest among us. He is macrobiotic.

Certainly, no single alternative approach to healing predominated. There were people who were into Reiki, or massage, or meditation, or diet, or vitamins. And frankly, most people did not stick with any one approach. There was a lot of walking around.

Virtually every long-term survivor was involved in the political struggle to end AIDS. My theory of why that might be so is that you can very easily be consumed by your AIDS. You can close yourself off from the world around you. It seems to be very important when you have AIDS, to get outside your own tragedy, to know that you are having an influence on other people. This activism seems to have a healing effect.

I have been pretty prominent in my opposition to the use of AZT. Although I didn't expect to find similar opposition among the long-term survivors, I did. It was pleasantly surprising. Of my four dozen survivors, only four had ever used it at all; and of those four, three are now dead and one is dying of AZT-induced lymphoma. The overwhelming majority of long-term survivors had somehow managed to resist the enormous pressure to take AZT. This was very much a distinguishing characteristic of long-term survivors: a skepticism about experimental medications. Long-term survivors, for what it's worth, take a very skeptical wait-and-see approach.

Nine out of 10 drugs that ever enter any phase of human testing fail, as either non-effective or too toxic. Well, that is quite startling if true: if the odds are stacked against you 9 to 1, then I do not understand the current drugs-into-body frenzy.[2] I believe that my AIDS activist friends who are in the forefront of this drugs-into-body frenzy are misleading people with AIDS, who are frightened and desperate. The activists only seem to talk about two possible outcomes to taking an experimental drug: one is that it works and the other is that it doesn't work. But there is a third, much more common possibility, which is that you will be worse off than if you did nothing at all. And nobody likes to talk about that. But from my reading of the literature, sometimes doing nothing is much better than doing the wrong thing. And it would seem, on the record of government-sponsored clinical trials, that most people are actually worse off taking these toxic drugs than if they hadn't taken them at all.

---

[2]"Drugs into bodies!" was an Act Up slogan.

CHAPTER X

Thinking Positive: The AIDS Cult and Its Seroconverts[1]

Ian Young

Purposely, the twenty-something boys, who have never known a sex life without AIDS, fatalistically expose themselves to HIV as a test of ritual manhood.

— Jack Fritscher, *Mapplethorpe: Assault with a Deadly Camera,* 1994.

Deliver me from blood gatherers, O God,
Thou art the God of my health.

— Book of Common Prayer

At the local gay bars and dance clubs, the raves and fetish nights and "AIDS fundraising" events, a new style of body ornament is becoming fashionable. Young gay men are beginning to sport tattoos, usually in block letters on the upper arm, that spell out HIV, followed by a minus sign. The idea, of course, is that when (when!) you seroconvert, you pay a follow-up visit to your tattooist, who changes your minus to a plus. Simple.

The convertible (one way only!) tattoos signal an unsettling phenomenon that is only now beginning to be acknowledged. An astonishing number of young gay men whose sexual activity began only after the implementation of the "Safe Sex" and "AIDS

[1]This essay has not previously been published.

Education" programs of the Eighties and Nineties, are seroconverting — testing Positive for HIV, the virus widely believed to cause AIDS. One estimate has it that one in three twenty-year old gay men will be HIV-infected or dead of AIDS by the age of thirty. Many of them, according to psychologist Walt Odets, not only recognize the possibility of AIDS for themselves, but "accept it as a destiny about which they can do very little."

A pair of recently published books, Odets' own *In the Shadow of the Epidemic: Being HIV Negative in the Age of AIDS*[2] and William I. Johnston's *HIV Negative: How the Uninfected Are Affected by AIDS*[3], explore this new insouciance about seroconversion and offer some disturbing insights into contemporary attitudes. Odets is a clinical psychologist and psychotherapist; Johnston is the facilitator of a discussion group for gay, HIV Negative men. Working independently, they have amassed considerable evidence of what Odets describes as "a psychological epidemic among uninfected gay men."

Now in its fifteenth year, the protracted AIDS crisis has had an impact on everyone in the gay community, uninfected and infected alike. Odets writes that he sees "innumerable examples of psychological problems among gay men that seven years ago would have been unusual and noteworthy, but are now so common that they pass almost without comment." Many gay men are afraid to become close to anyone, as either lover or friend, for fear any intimate involvement will be terminated by

---

[2]Walt Odets, *In the Shadow of the Epidemic: Being HIV Negative in the Age of AIDS*, Durham, N.C., Duke University Press, 1995.

[3]William I. Johnston, *HIV Negative: How the Uninfected Are Affected by AIDS*, N.Y., Plenum Press, 1995.

early death. As one man put it, "I've never thought about having a relationship for more than a couple of years, because I've never dated anyone who was going to live longer than that."

Odets' and Johnston's books are the latest additions to a growing body of literature documenting the complex varieties of "survivor guilt" now experienced by increasing numbers of uninfected gay men. Both authors discuss the finding that in today's breezy, out-of-the-closet gay ghetto, HIV Negative men tend to be profoundly clinically depressed, anxious, disoriented, hypochondriacal, uncertain about the future, sexually dysfunctional, deeply demoralized and psychically numb. Many abuse alcohol or drugs, and their physicians prescribe them millions of dollars worth of tranquillizers, sleeping pills, anti-depressants and sedatives every year. More and more uninfected men, Odets finds, now "live in nearly every detail like a dying man — disoriented, piecemeal, and with no assumption of a future."

From his years of intensive talks with friends, patients and discussion group clients, Odets concludes that this widespread, endemic depression has its origins not only in reactions to the current health crisis, but also in "a destructive mix of old developmental problems" that have usually begun in childhood. Substance abuse is often chronic, reflecting mood disorders, loneliness and stress; in this, HIV Negative gay men probably differ little from their HIV Positive brothers. We may now be starting to recognize longstanding patterns of psychoimmune disturbance in a second generation of gay men — a generation that has come to sexual awareness during the AIDS era.

A few years ago, when conservative commentator William F. Buckley, Jr. suggested that PWAs should all be forcibly tattooed (on the arm and/or the buttocks) for instant recognition, there was widespread disgust at the idea and embarrassment that the apparently urbane Buckley would suggest it. Now, such tattooing is available on a voluntary basis and there is no lack of takers. After a decade of propaganda about Safe Sex, a sizeable cohort of young men becomes eligible every year for HIV+ tattoos. Bill Buckley's American Auschwitz Theme Park is almost here, and no boxcars will be required.

One effect of the ubiquitous official warnings about "risk behavior" and "vectors of (AIDS) transmission", is that more and more gay men now believe their body fluids to be dangerous, and "define certain behaviors, such as anal sex or oral sex, as *unsafe in and of themselves,* without regard to whether one of the people involved had HIV." "It is common," writes Odets, "for gay men now to say that anal sex is 'unsafe' even when practised by two HIV-negative people." William S. Burroughs is fond of quoting one survey that found most people believe you can get AIDS from anal intercourse, whether or not HIV is present.

Anxieties about gayness, and about intimacy, now frequently express themselves as fear of viral contamination, providing an ostensibly rational reason to avoid what has always been problematic. When HIV is identified with feared (and unconsciously desired) homosexual intimacy, the result is a powerful draw toward seroconversion. The uninfected men interviewed in both these books repeatedly express the view that HIV Positives live richer, more complex, more "authentic" lives, get more attention, are better able to take risks — including, significantly, the "risk of intimacy" — and that only with such risk-taking can life be meaningful and full.

This perceived link between HIV Positive status and emotional fulfillment is just one among many factors now propelling gay men toward seroconversion. These pressures emanate from the AIDS Establishment's group assumptions about gay men, assumptions which are more and more clearly reflected in the ghettoized gay community itself. And it is the power and diversity of the pressures to seroconvert that constitute the central, disturbing message of both these books.

After the Reagan administration pronounced in 1984 that HIV was the sole cause of AIDS, lucrative patents on HIV-antibody tests were granted to leading AIDS researchers, and aggressive promotion of HIV-antibody testing began. At first, most gay and AIDS advocacy groups considered testing to be dangerous and oppressive. In the mid-Eighties, people entering the "Test Sites" (a term eerily reminiscent of "nuclear test sites") often had to make their way through lines of vocal gay demonstrators. Governments and pharmaceutical companies then directed a light dusting of money to selected recipients and the protests died down. Soon a broad consensus developed that testing was a virtue, a civic duty, and the smart thing to do.

Testing Positive, in the current wisdom, leads to "early intervention", by which is meant the administration of large quantities of pharmaceutical products — the so-called "antivirals" — principally nucleoside analogues, whose devastating "side-effects" often replicate AIDS symptoms. Whether subsequent illnesses are caused by the inevitable "progress" of the virus, or by a self-fulfilling prophecy is debatable.

The quotations and first-person accounts by HIV Negative men in these studies suggest that while an HIV Positive test result was originally looked upon as a calamity, this is no longer always the case. This is partly because some PWAs are learning how to take care of themselves and are living longer, and partly because a growing number of gay men see HIV infection and subsequent AIDS not as something that can or should be avoided, but as, in Johnston's words, something "fundamentally linked to gay identity". Certainly it has been represented to them that way. Heterosexuals and lesbians are told, "AIDS doesn't discriminate!" But gay men have come to perceive it as an inextricable part of their "community", their "identity", and their future. One female-to-male transsexual told his therapist that his transformation to a gay man would only be complete when he had contracted HIV! I have heard gay men repeat the homophobic joke: "GAY stands for Got AIDS Yet?".

In the Seventies and early Eighties, a ghettoized consumerism (fast food, fast drugs, fast sex, quick-fix medicine) was packaged and sold as "the Gay Lifestyle". Now AIDS is increasingly presented as the new Gay Lifestyle. In the gay community of the Nineties, everything revolves around AIDS.

This AIDS-centered vision of community life has even encroached on lesbian society. In 1994, after the founder of the British organization for lesbians with HIV, Positive Strength, revealed that her claim to seropositive status was false, AIDS activist Simon Watney spoke of "an imaginary epidemic [of] fantasy AIDS" among British lesbians. Lesbian writer Robin Gorna wrote that "although there are many gay men who also lie about their HIV status, it seems that some lesbians feel unable to articulate their own issues alongside the horror of AIDS. If you are a young dyke, your identity is all tied up with AIDS, yet it's not your stuff." She added that there was no evidence to suggest lesbian sex poses any significant AIDS risk: lesbians with AIDS, she said, tend to contract it from drug use and/or sex with men, which she described as "still a taboo subject in the lesbian community."[4] In all the fracas about how many lesbians get

---

[4]Trish Lesslie, "Out in England: Lesbian AIDS Envy?" in *Out*, October 1994, pp. 26-27.

AIDS, Gorna's remark that many gay men lie about having HIV seems to have been overlooked.

Walt Odets draws our attention to the attitude, widespread in the gay community, that only PWAs and HIV Positives have a right to express strong feelings. He recalls that when he voiced his concerns about the emotional well-being of HIV Negative gay men, he found it was considered inappropriate for HIV Negatives to "experience feelings about their own lives worthy of discussion or worthy of the concern and attention of others." The feelings of those regarded as "uninfected" are widely felt to be "selfish, inappropriate, or simply ridiculous." Often, HIV Negatives are even seen as The Enemy; one man, on the steering committee of a "mental health" conference, when told of an HIV Negative discussion group, retorted, "That's like Germans getting together ... to congratulate themselves on not being Jewish!"

Society has never made the well-being of gay men a priority. On the other hand, if you have AIDS or are HIV Positive, a range of social services, support groups, medical benefits and other perks becomes immediately available. Suddenly, attention is paid. Variations of the same phrase crop up again and again in the sentimental AIDS literature: "I never knew how much I was loved until I got AIDS." It makes a great ad slogan, if AIDS is what you're selling.

In the urban gay ghettos of the Eighties and Nineties, a whole AIDS Culture has emerged — an "AIDS Community" based on an ever-shifting mélange of medical and subcultural assumptions. This new blood brotherhood is beginning to form a kind of Inner Order within the exoteric conglomeration of the lesbian and gay scene, and a growing number of glossy magazines now devote themselves to the perks and pleasures of the Positive Lifestyle. And one "comes out" into this Lifestyle in one way only: by seroconverting. Seroconversion is the ritual that all who would join the cult must endure. Those who have lost friends, or, especially, one or more lovers, to AIDS may claim honorary membership. The cult's unofficial badge of honor is a looped red ribbon, usually pinned to the chest, or rather to the coat. Originally a fund-raising favor, the "red ribbon" is now commercially available in many stylish designer forms: one can choose from ceramic, dyed leather, or 24 karat gold encrusted with red stones. Elizabeth Taylor is one of the few who can afford a diamond and ruby "ribbon". Of course, fashion is fickle and the red ribbon is already coming to be regarded as somewhat passé, not to say kitsch.

Under the pressure of protracted crisis, the transformation of signals, policies and identities has been relentless. In the Eighties and early Nineties, the figure of the AIDS activist, the seething ACT UP clone, body pumped under the white political T-shirt, head shaved, concentration-camp style, became, for a while, a symbol of erotic resonance, a sexual icon. Having exhausted itself in unfocused anger, the fashion is less popular now than it was.

The ongoing roster of AIDS dead (lots of blank space left on that memorial, how thoughtful) constitutes the raison d'être of this new, prototypically postmodern, community. Obituaries and funerals are its social glue; its chief dramatic form is the memorial service. Every two weeks, when the new issue of *Xtra!* comes out, everyone turns to the obituaries first. The Toronto version of this Canadian gay newspaper combine (for it has cloned itself) publishes an annual roster of AIDS dead, under the banner headline "Proud Lives." Deaths from non-AIDS-related causes are relegated to a separate, less prominent, section bearing the mundane and rather dismissive tag, "Other Losses." HIV Positive decedents are sometimes placed in the "Proud Lives" section, even if they committed suicide or fell off a mountain. If you're Positive, there's only one way to die, and we're going to hold you to it.

The overshadowing of all other gay issues by the AIDS agenda (first pointed out by Darrell Yates Rist), and the frequent dismissal of HIV Negative concerns, has generated widespread feelings of "disenfranchisement" among uninfected gay men. These feelings are reinforced when the uninfected are told to behave *as if* they were infected: "Be good. Have Safe Sex" — even if they are in a monogamous relationship with an uninfected partner! Walt Odets suggests that these injunctions have been ineffective in promoting safer sex, as well as psychologically disastrous.

Within the urban gay community, the uninfected now constitute what William Johnston calls a "psychic minority" — one that appears increasingly eager to Think Positive and join the psychic majority, the HIV Community. Though it would have been inconceivable only a few years ago, a Positive HIV antibody test result, or even an AIDS diagnosis, now frequently results in a *decrease* in anxiety! The director of one health service agency reports that crisis responses requiring urgent counselling were generated by Negative test results at a three-to-one margin over Positive ones!

Among the responses to being told of a Negative test result: "All my friends are Positive — how can I relate to them?" "Everyone's going to be very angry at me." "I feel like I'm being left out of the great event of our time." "I hoped I would be Positive so it would give me an excuse to go back out and drink and drug." "I feel as if I won't really have come out until I'm HIV Positive." "It's a lot simpler to think about AIDS than about being gay." "Guys who get AIDS get a lot more attention." And, my own favorite, "Shit! I'm going to have to go to work tomorrow after all."

One gay man told me recently that when he revealed to an acquaintance that he was HIV Negative, he received the sneering (presumably rhetorical) reply, "How come? Didn't anyone want your tired old ass?" A gay student, who was relieved at his Negative test results, nevertheless made a wryly revealing comment about the whole process and everyone's attitudes to it: "For once," he said, "I was glad I failed a test."

One contributor to Johnston's book describes a gay man who eventually seroconverted after many attempts: he "had a beatific glow on his face when he found out he was Positive. He had been expecting this for so long, and finally the desired outcome was achieved." (His lover, he feared, was about to "dump" him if he remained stubbornly Negative.) This new attitude — utterly unforseen by the pundits of AIDS Education or its consumers — leads Odets to ask whether counsellors "unconsciously suggest that a Positive test result is more 'important' than a Negative (one)?" The language used suggests they do; certainly they focus almost exclusively on preparing their clients for "Positive" results.

The man with the beatific glow is one of a growing group of gay men who see their "progress" (this is the official term[5]) to seroconversion and to AIDS as somehow desirable or inevitable. For the burgeoning cohort of seroconverts, the assumption of HIV Positive identity has become an important rite of passage in their lives as gay men. A beatific glow is a characteristic feature of religious conversion experiences, and in many ways, these men resemble the freshly inducted members of a cult.

---

[5]In scientific circles, HIV Positives who remain healthy are referred to as "non-progressors".

There is a growing perception that for a gay man today to be HIV Positive is, well, *positive.* Connotations as fundamental as those suggested by the words "positive" and "negative" are deeply imbedded in our interpretations of the terminology we use. People do not easily transpose black and white, or accept a Positive result as Negative. Nor can the frequent use of the word "status" be considered inconsequential; we are lectured about our antibody "status", the subliminal suggestion being that testing Positive, becoming "Body Positive", and adopting a "positive attitude" involves gaining a positive status, becoming worthy of concern.[6] The phenomena of the courageous, Positive seroconvert and his neurotic, Negative twin have evolved out of the bizarre, dogmatic logic of HIV fundamentalism — what Walt Odets calls the "contradictions, inconsistencies and anomalies" of AIDS.

Odets writes that "a return to unprotected sex among gay men after about 1988 is now widely recognized." Why in 1988, four years after the announcement of HIV as the cause of AIDS? My own experience from periodic visits to New York City, an AIDS epicenter, is that the years 1987 to 1988 constituted the height of what the novelist Andrew Holleran has succinctly called "The Fear". Christopher Street was emptier than it has ever been and many gay men were afraid even to kiss. Protracted, inhibited grief and paralyzing terror seemed, even to a visitor, to be causing all sorts of neuroses and a kind of mass mental break-

---

[6]This may be doubly so for those addicted to intravenous drugs, who are now said to comprise the majority of new PWAs (though the periodically changing definition of the syndrome makes reliable statistics impossible to assemble). In the inner cities, those who want to abandon their heroin habit can ask to have their names added to a list; it may be months or years before they become eligible for a daily ration of methadone.

down. If the "return to unprotected sex" began in the late Eighties as Odets believes, it may well have begun as a reactive symptom of that breakdown — an heroic defiance of fear by stoically embracing what was believed to be inevitable.

As the AIDS crisis was about to begin, the poet and novelist George Whitmore wrote that we engaged in so many of our "rebellious" acts (like crawling around on all fours on the floor of the Mineshaft at four in the morning, or participating in the dangerous sexual scenes that had become so popular) to show that we could do these things "without flinching" — that we were not, after all, sissies. John Rechy endowed sexually promiscuous gay men with "heroic" qualities, calling them the shock troops of the sexual revolution. Is the same defensive need to prove one's masculinity, one's courage, and one's "in group" status now helping to create the phenomenon of the seroconvert?

Survivor guilt often involves the feeling that one should not have survived — and the hope that one *will not* survive. The urban gay lifestyle is designed for youth, and for those committed to that lifestyle, the loss of youth may seem more terrible than a fatal illness. Michelangelo Signorile wrote in a recent column[7] that "far too many gay men say they actually fear growing old in a gay world that puts the young and buffed on a pedestal while treating the over-35 crowd like lepers." He tells of one young guy who has unsafe sex because "he doesn't want to live to be 50. He doesn't want to be another aging queen, being jeered at by people like himself." Another man said he felt

---

[7]Michelangelo Signorile, "Unsafe Like Me" in *Out*, October 1994, p. 24. Signorile argues that "safer sex has broken down substantially.... It is time for drastic approaches and lots of self-examination. Our sexual culture is often *not* liberating.... And we must change it."

so "beneath" the men he was attracted to that he'd "do anything" for them, including have unsafe sex.

Walt Odets concludes that "for some, the self-destructive aspects of unprotected sex are important incentives to practise it." This, he emphasizes, "has nothing to do with complacency, nor will traditional AIDS education address it."

The AIDS System now entrenched in the urban gay ghettos has aggressively promoted HIV antibody testing ("the AIDS test"), and most available AIDS Education has been oriented toward encouraging people — particularly gay men — to "get tested." Former presidential candidate Bruce Babbitt described the system as a "voodoo health policy" animated by the idea that "if we keep sticking needles into people and taking blood tests, the disease will go away." The apparent non sequitur only begins to make sense if, unconsciously, it is not so much the disease but the seropositives who are being wished away, with the AIDS System constructed as a wish-fulfillment around the group fantasy, and camouflaged as medical services.

"There are two ways to find out", read a slogan on the outside of an envelope one gay man received in the mail: "You can get tested. Or you can get sick." Even though AIDS was nowhere mentioned, he "knew right away what this cryptic message meant." It felt, he said, "like an assault". The letter was from Project Inform, a group that began as a dissident AIDS advocacy group and devolved into what one commentator called a "power broker, coordinating sections of the AIDS industry with the appropriate government agencies." In a letter to the gay paper, the *San Francisco Sentinel,* one reader described Project Inform as a "pharmaceutical pimp".

Extensive sections of Johnson's *HIV Negative* are contributed by various "uninfected" gay men, some identified, others using pseudonyms. And Odets' book, the more analytic of the two, contains many briefer quotes drawn from the author's extensive counselling experience. Among the remarks: "Negative men are like my family: they have no feelings." "What I know is that I am going to follow my heart, and I think it's leading me to the (kind of) understanding that having HIV gives a person." "They will have a cure for it by the time we get it." Another remark I have heard repeatedly is: "If I test Positive, I can start taking care of myself."

There is a common feeling that to try to stay Negative — to "struggle" to stay Negative, as one man put it — is simply too difficult, too destructive of any joy in life. This is hardly surprising when the rules of "safe" behavior are at once so stringent and so slippery. Is oral sex safe? Is rimming with a dental dam OK and if it is, why should we want to do it? Should I worry about that sharp pizza crust that might cut my lip and let the virus in? Am I condemned to stay around and watch all my friends die?

In the shadow of such conundrums, becoming Positive seems to some like a doorway to intimacy, light and love, and life with AIDS, for all its horrors, begins to appear more rewarding, or just simpler, than life without it. Whatever the respective merits of these questions, the mental soil in which they grow is fertile ground for a Positive choice.

Eric Rofes of the National Gay and Lesbian Task Force, who provides an introduction to *HIV Negative*, describes himself and other uninfected gay men, the "population of supposed survivors", as people "left to walk the earth like robots or zombies, telling ourselves and others that everything's fine while we are actually numb, cut off from our emotions." This contrasts vividly with the dark, vampiric glamour of AIDS. Walt Odets refers to "the appeal of illness." All these attitudes fuel the desire to seroconvert.

Another common observation made of HIV testing is that testees often doubt or question their Negative results, but seldom their Positive ones. The psychologist Rachel Schochet found that the more bereavements men had experienced, the more they tended to doubt their own Negative status — and the more they engaged in unprotected sex.

This doubting of Negative results is built into the administration of the testing system itself. Positive results, we are told (falsely), are never wrong, but Negative results may be "premature" or "false Negatives", or unreflective of the virus' supposed "window of opportunity". And so when we test Negative, we are encouraged to restrain our relief, and to return regularly to the Test Site. If we did not keep coming back like a yo-yo, presumably we would snap our strings and go careening off, cavalierly spreading HIV around, to ourselves or to others, Typhoid Mary off on a bender. In fact, the AIDS System, by failing to support thoughtful self-knowledge, and by subliminally suggesting that a Positive outcome is inevitable and desirable, encourages the very behavior it ostensibly seeks to prevent. The constant state of anxiety it instills damages both the mental faculties and the immune system.

The HIV antibody test (usually called "the HIV test" or "the AIDS test") is surrounded by an enormous amount of stress, with unfortunate immunological consequences. "Paul Fielding", a pseudonymous gay man quoted by Johnston, makes the point: "You weren't supposed to have stress, because stress could destroy your T-cells.... So you had to try to smile living in a pressure cooker."

Warnings about "risk groups" and "risk behaviors" strike a profoundly ambiguous note in a society where risk is associated with entrepreneurial behavior, glamorous chance-taking and competition, and is highly valued. Risking danger has always provided a test of manhood for rebellious youth: practising "unsafe sex" is a challenge, a way of accepting a dare, a contemporary version of the "chicken run" depicted in *Rebel Without a Cause.*

The French writer Hervé Guibert, wrote of his lover Muzil, who routinely visited the baths for sex, in spite of his poor health. Muzil remarked that

> The baths have never been more popular, and now they're fantastic. The danger lurking everywhere has created new complicities, new tenderness, new solidarities. Before, no one ever said a word; now we talk to one another. We all know exactly whey we're there.[8]

The "danger lurking" is of course the demonized "AIDS virus" whose alleged propensity for "lurking", "hiding", and other "clever" behavior is said to explain the many cases of HIV Negative AIDS. And the men are there to live dangerously.

Pervasive pressure to seroconvert has produced the phenomenon of the compulsive repeat tester, the uninfected individual who is caught on a "testing treadmill", making frequent visits to a Test Site, or to several Test Sites ("Is it a good lab?") and always doubting Negative results. Johnston discusses an attempt in Boston to start a discussion group for such compulsive

---

[8]Hervé Guibert, *To the Friend Who Did Not Save My Live,* New York, Atheneum, 1991, pp. 21-22.

retesters. "The group didn't work, because they all wanted individual attention.... They didn't want their story to compete with anybody else's, because their story was the most important." A compulsive need for attention is easily met by the ministrations of the AIDS industry, which is set up to provide all the attention needed, once seroconversion is achieved. The compulsive retester is a seroconvert in the making.

The much vaunted Safe Sex and AIDS Education programs of the Eighties and Nineties have been a spectacular failure. They are as counterproductive as the campaign against unmarried teenage pregnancies in the Black community — and for the same reason: the underlying causes of the phenomena remain unaddressed.

In my own city, Toronto, promiscuous unsafe sex is a popular feature of the bathhouses which have been springing up again over the past few years. Some of them are now licensed to sell beer, which they supplement, unofficially, with poppers and crack cocaine (smoke it in your room) as additional perks. Here too, the rate of seroconversion among young men — and subsequent entry into the ramshackle labyrinth of the AIDS System — is climbing. And *Xtra's* obituary column isn't getting any smaller.

It is becoming apparent that the actual consequences of the AIDS System are at variance with its stated aims. There are unconscious factors at play here — unidentified, even unacknowledged. As Eric Rofes says in his Foreword: "Something is happening to us which no-one wants to face."

Odets explains how the AIDS System's current approach to prevention is modelled on a "public health/social marketing model" composed of relentless propaganda ("Information and Education") and the utilization of what he delicately describes as "selected community leaders" to mold group behavior. Complex psychosocial issues are avoided; feelings about sex and death, personal worth, goals, intimacy and human needs remain for the most part unexplored outside a relatively few independent therapy groups. Its simplistic strategy is based on the assumptions that sex for gay men is merely a mechanical procedure without human meaning, and that immune suppression can be contracted only through intimate contact with the blood or semen of an "infected" partner. (Public concerns about saliva, tears and sweat are occasionally expressed, but so far have been fairly successfully dismissed.)[9]

The nature of the relationship of HIV to AIDS has been a subject of fierce dispute, though the debate has been rather one-sided: the skeptics (who include a scattering of scientists and three Nobel prizewinners) present detailed critiques, which the HIV fundamentalists either ignore or respond to with abuse.[10] If, as seems increasingly likely, HIV turns out not to be the sole cause of AIDS, every AIDS Education program on the continent will have to be rethought from the ground up and some people might even be cleaning out their desks. Naturally, critiques of HIV dogma are vehemently resisted by the growing army of HIV support staff.

---

[9]A recent issue of *Poz,* a slick magazine aimed at HIV Positive gay men, includes an article on a new, saliva-based antibody test, a "plastic stick held between the cheek and gum for two minutes". On the following page, a separate article informs readers that it is the presence of a protease inhibitor that prevents the detection or transmission of HIV through saliva.

[10]For a summary of dissident views on HIV's role in AIDS, see Neville Hodgkinson, *AIDS: The Failure of Contemporary Science,* London, Fourth Estate, 1996.

The question of how Positive results are achieved seems equally problematic. HIV Positive test results have frequently registered in individuals who have been exposed to certain other pathogens such as malaria, or who have suffered a recent bout of influenza. The current tests, it seems, are not as specific as they might be. A ground-breaking paper from Australia, published in *Bio/Technology* in June of 1993, demonstrated that the favored "AIDS tests" fail three basic criteria: they are not specific, there is no standard interpretation, and their results are not reproducible.[11]

In addition, several series of research experiments have shown that under certain conditions, lab animals may develop antibodies to parts of HIV without ever having been in contact with the virus. When some animals in a group were exposed to viruses and developed antibodies, other, unexposed, animals in the same "cohort" also began to test Positive.[12] Could gay men, too, be developing antibody Positive status in resonance with already infected members of their Cohort? If so, it might help to explain the increasing number of "anomalous seroconversions" now being reported.

The issue of drugs (both legal and illegal) provides another example of poorly examined assumptions generating a dangerously simplistic approach. Official AIDS education literature almost always warns that recreational drugs may "impair judgment" and so "lead to unsafe sex", but the health risks and immunosuppressive qualities of many drugs are seldom mentioned. In the absence of community-based programs to counter heroin use, we

[11]See Papadopulos-Eleopulos *et al.*, Appendix A.

[12]See Ian Young, *The Stonewall Experiment*, Cassell, 1995, pp. 253-256.

are simply urged to bleach, and never share, the hygienically wrapped needles distributed by AIDS organizations. Many physicians regard drugs and alcohol as "coping mechanisms" and sanction their abuse by gay patients, Negative and Positive. Kicking a drinking or drug habit, like giving up promiscuous sex, is seen as a near impossibility for gay men, and substance abuse programs (particularly if peer-run) are often regarded as threatening to the doctor-patient relationship.

The version of public health marketing that has come to dominate AIDS Education is patterned on a model for the treatment of addictive/compulsive disorders. This is hardly surprising, as the medical establishment has traditionally assumed that gay men necessarily regard sex as a mechanical process without deeper meaning. Educational proposals that attempt to address spiritual matters are dismissed as unrealistic. Inquiry into the *reasons* for addictive/compulsive behavior would entail an examination of socioeconomic pressures, motivations and group beliefs — and is usually ruled out as too difficult, too dangerous or too expensive.

We encourage what we assume. The current AIDS System fosters the addictive/compulsive psychology that social beliefs ascribe to gay men. Group behavior is then played out according to social expectations, alternating between two phases representing control and release.

The compulsive, Control phase involves strict abstinence or avoidance — in this case, rigid adherence to the proclaimed principles of Safe Sex, which are presented as unclear, yet essential — even when there is no apparent reason for them, as with sex between Negative partners. This attitude generates tension, confusion, demoralization and suspicion.

In the second, addictive, Release phase, the restrictive psychic controls become too stressful and collapse into a "slip" or "binge", involving deliberate self-exposure to HIV and other pathogens, often under the influence of immunosuppressive substances and mental states. Attempts are made to prevent, minimize, postpone or substitute for the Release phase. But such simplistic attempts at enforcing control (whether by propaganda or legal injunctions) rarely work, and when they fail, guilt feelings are reinforced. The notorious failure of most "diet" plans provides a typical example.

One of Odets' most astute insights is that social organizations often act as containers for forbidden feelings. Shared, organizationally approved feelings are substituted for genuine ones; emotional impoverishment is masked, and anger repressed. Rather than encouraging thoughtfulness and understanding on the part of gay men, current AIDS Education programs have insisted on politically correct scripts, placing us in the familiar role of dependent children.

Odets sees HIV Positive gay men as allowing themselves to be cast in the role of the "needy" child in a family, with HIV Negative men assuming the role of the resentful, "needless" child, desperate for his share of attention from parental figures. If the sick sibling is perceived as getting all the attention, one solution is to become sick oneself. The metaphor of gay men as children or perpetual juveniles has been common and pervasive; even gay protesters have adopted it: "acting up" is, after all, what children do to get attention.[13]

---

[13]In 1992, The Act Up chapter in Chicago split into two factions, one for HIV Positive people, the other for HIV Negatives. The possibility that a member might not know his "status" was presumably unthinkable.

And there is something else going on here. The growing ranks of seroconverts are approaching the seroconversion process as an opportunity for something that young men, and especially young gay men, in our society, desperately need — an initiatory rite of passage.

Our society's ideology is a consumerist one, and its rituals tend to be the vapid pseudo-activities of consumerism — shopping, smoking, television watching, package holidays. But rites of passage (coming of age, for example) demand a special kind of ritual to mark the transition from one psychological and social state to another. Apart from the melancholy duties of draft and voter registration, the only such rituals now generally available to young men involve the acquisition of a driver's license and a first car (either purchased or stolen).

Rites of passage signal the ritual death of the old self and a symbolic rebirth into a new identity, accepted and honored by the community. For young gay men, "coming out" once served this function, but as secrecy about being gay has lessened and sexual categories are blurring, coming out has become less meaningful and unsettlingly inconclusive. For the most part, significant gay rites of passage have simply been unavailable. Instead, we are offered rituals of addiction and compulsion, which we adopt as our own. Seroconversion fills the need for a gay rite of passage in the Nineties.

Journalist and AIDS dissident Celia Farber has aptly called HIV "a demon, which we worship with our terror" and attempt to placate with buildings, organizations, conferences, and global programs. No such cult can continue for over a decade without developing its own forms of ritual obeisance, and the AIDS system has proved to be no exception.

The HIV testing ceremony is highly ritualized, demanding a visit to a special, rather fearsome place — a sacred place, the Test Site — with priests and acolytes in attendance: the various physicians, psychiatrists, social workers, peer counsellors and AIDS workers hovering or bustling about, many wearing their white robes of office.

The ceremony involves a literal blood sacrifice, drawn with a hypodermic needle by a nurse or paramedic. Some initiates faint. It is accompanied by highly structured readings from sacred texts: AIDS Education and Safe Sex scripts. It incorporates a Time of Trial — the stressful period of several days or weeks involved in waiting for one's results. During this time, one's thoughts are concentrated almost continuously on HIV as the shared object of fear and devotion. And — if the test is passed, if the results are Positive — one is embraced into the community with new status, HIV Positive status, and increased attention. One enters the AIDS System, "the AIDS Community".

The very way we look at the phenomenon of AIDS has its psychological consequences. Belief in HIV as the cause of AIDS has led not only to a vast, self-perpetuating AIDS industry, but to the establishment of a medico-religious cult.

A recent issue of a Canadian gay magazine contained a news item about a Toronto gay man, Sean Martin, who had been diagnosed as HIV Positive.[14] A year later, a second test reversed the verdict, and Martin is quoted as saying that though the HIV Positive friends he had made were "very nice to me about it", telling them he was Negative was one of the toughest things he'd ever done. He couldn't help feeling that he was "abandon-

[14]"HIV Negative Guilt" in *Wayves*, October 1995, p. 13.

ing" them, he said, and his new status made him feel he was "breaking the faith".

In his classic study of modern initiatory behaviors, the psychologist Luigi Zoja writes: "The archetypal need to transcend one's present state at any cost ... is especially strong in those who find themselves in a state of meaninglessness, lacking both a sense of identity and a precise social role."[15] This description would appear to fit many of the men interviewed in Odets' and Johnson's books; it is particularly applicable to seroconverts.

The gay health crisis has reached a stage in which seroconversion is becoming institutionalized as the most important rite of passage in the life of a gay man. Significantly, its place in consumer society is a paradoxical one. The seroconvert, the young gay man who "chooses Positive" and adopts the Positive Lifestyle is, like the drug addict, someone who participates in the social ritual, but denies the dominant social imperative — to be a "responsible" economic being. His Positive status gives him the permission and the means to solve one of the perennial problems of youth — how to conform and rebel at the same time.

In his consideration of drugs and ritual, Zoja points out that in our society, the addict "is not absent from the economic picture, but rather present in a destructive way."[16] The seroconvert is also motivated to be "present in a destructive way". He drops out of the workaday world to live on disability or viatical benefits — income predicated on the assumption, the tacit agreement, that he will soon die. And after he "progresses" to

---

[15]Luigi Zoja, *Drugs, Addiction and Initiation: The Modern Search for Ritual*, Sigo Press, 1989, p. 15.

[16]Zoja, *op. cit.*, p. 14.

"full-blown AIDS" he is even more "present in a destructive way".[17]

This suicide by degrees, abetted by so many forces, is the latest manifestation of the idea of the Homosexual as Sacrificial Victim, unconsciously embodying remnants of ancient themes of ritual sacrifice. The Sacrificial Victim has finally become aware of his role, but not yet able to slough it off, has begun to accede to it with some degree of deliberation. The seroconvert sets out to prove himself worthy of the sacrificial ritual, the testing, that he undergoes. This quest exemplifies what Zoja calls the "negative sacrifice, where only the destructive part of the act survives, and which is carried out by that person we call a negative hero." Of course, there is a positive side as well. The afflicted homosexual also becomes a "cross carrier", taking onto himself a complex of rejected and projected group feelings, fears and impulses. With his death, all these are, temporarily, exorcised.

---

[17]Viatical settlement companies purchase the life insurance policies of people who are believed to be terminally sick. Many of their advertisements exploit the theme of immediate gratification — for example, one of the 20 viatical settlement ads in the July 1996 issue of *POZ Magazine* states:

> Turn your LIFE INSURANCE into CASH, NOW CASH NOW, CASH NOW, CASH NOW, CASH NOW, CASH NOW, CASH NOW, CASH NOW ...
>
> Your NEEDS must be met.................. NOW
> Your DREAMS must be fulfilled........ NOW.
>
> [Capitalization as in original ad.]

Another viatical settlement ad in a gay newspaper included a testimonial from a satisfied client, who said he had been able to buy "the car of my dreams", and who made the important point, "It didn't even interfere with my benefits." In other words, the viatical settlement money did not prevent him from receiving his usual welfare, disability, and other "benefits".

In the classic pattern of initiation, desire for the death of the old self is followed by symbolic rebirth and the welcoming of the new self into the community of initiated peers. In the self-sacrifice of the seroconvert, this process is inverted: the old, negative self, rather than being overcome and sloughed off, is incorporated, with all its negativity, into the new self, who, instead of being enriched with new life, assumes new burdens of guilt and early death — burdens which novels, movies and folklore have long projected onto the figure of the Homosexual.

Seroconversion induces both the expectation of a short life and the feeling that one's desirability as a lover is diminished. It is a combination that frequently leads to the feeling: I'm dying and no-one will want me, so I may as well party with whatever short time I have left. And so the party becomes a Dance of Death. In his book *The Savage Garden,* the novelist and diarist Paul Reed muses that many of his friends:

> have resumed a life that is in many ways similar to the life we pursued a decade ago — the gym, an afternoon rest ... the clubs.... The difference is that we now no longer work to pay the bills, we simply collect our disability checks. And we no longer feel that this is the beginning of a hot, fast life. It may be the last party, the final fling.[18]

In the Nineties, that final, AIDS-related "fling" has become both a phobia and a macabre obsession. One gay club in Manhattan recently hosted a creepy and popular new event called "Res-Erection", which consisted of a go-go boy feigning death in a

---

[18]Paul Reed, *The Savage Garden: A Journal,* House of Lillian, 1994, p. 14.

pseudo-Victorian setting while "horny revelers circled him and felt him up." *Très fin de siècle!*

It is becoming painfully evident that the AIDS Establishment's overt admonition to gay men to stay healthy is proving less effective than its subliminal inducements to seroconvert, and enter a system predicated on early death. Old assumptions about the homosexual's social status as scapegoat and victim are easily assimilated by the "victim culture" of the Nineties, which encourages troubled individuals to seek relief from their problems by adopting the role of irresponsible victim — conferred by illness, addiction or past abuse.

It is curious that the authors of both these studies apparently adhere to the belief that, in Odets' words, "a quirk of nature and timing has brought this epidemic to gay communities." One can only wonder which epidemic is being referred to. AIDS? Or the "psychological epidemic" that has grown up alongside it? Or are these concurrent epidemics merely aspects of the same overall pattern of psychoimmune disturbance — with the same underlying psychic, socioeconomic and environmental causes?

The health crisis in the gay community did not begin with the onset of AIDS in 1981; it was preceded by many years of psychological disturbance and chronic depression, reactions to a homophobia that was endemic and corrosive. In the Seventies, the already high instance of alcoholism and venereal disease among gay men was compounded by epidemics of drug abuse, hepatitis and intestinal parasites. By the first notices of what would come to be called AIDS, the immune systems of most men living "the Gay Lifestyle" had already been severely compromised.

In the early Nineties, the psychohistorian, medical researcher and AIDS activist Casper Schmidt described a shared sequence of psychoimmunological events in the gay men who develop AIDS. Their immune disturbances, he found, began with chronic depression, rooted in childhood unhappiness and related to socially induced guilt, internalized homophobia and a protracted "fight or flight" syndrome. As these feelings somatized into the body, the result was a chronically increased level of cortisol production, a steady depletion of T-cells, frantic overproduction of antibodies, and eventual immune collapse.

The evidence presented by Johnston and Odets suggests a continuation of this pattern, with the ominous difference that now, with the phenomenon of the seroconvert, gay men's identification of illness and early death as their destiny has moved more fully into group consciousness. Accepting the subliminal logic of HIV fundamentalism, gay men are beginning to see seroconversion and entry into the AIDS System as a gesture of solidarity with their fellows, a rite of passage, and a political act.

It is unlikely that anyone with a strong sense of self-worth would deliberately seek to seroconvert. But for a gay man who has internalized the negative judgements placed on him by family and society, it may well be "a lot simpler to think about [having] AIDS than about being gay." The film *Interview with the Vampire,* a work replete with coded references to a variety of contemporary fears (euthanasia, AIDS, immigration, gay families) contains the telling line: "If you think you deserve to die and you don't kill yourself, that makes you evil." To many, the evil of AIDS seems preferable to the perceived evil of living as a homosexual. AIDS itself may be horrible, but contracting AIDS is a relatively easy — and pleasurable — form of suicide.

AIDS today is not what it was in the early Eighties when the term was coined to avoid the embarrassing acronym GRID — Gay Related Immune Disorder. The definition has changed:

illnesses which were once considered key AIDS symptoms are now excluded if HIV is discovered not to be present; even the official record now lists well over 4,000 such cases. Pelvic inflammatory disorder in women may now result in an AIDS diagnosis if HIV is shown or assumed to be present. T-cell counts, ignored in the early years of AIDS, are now combined with the ever-changing list of disorders to produce diagnoses on a "one from column A, two from column B" basis. Pneumocystis carinii, long considered a protozoon, is now acknowledged to be a fungus. Consensus is growing that Kaposi's sarcoma, once regarded as a hallmark of AIDS in gay men, is not caused by HIV, and investigations into a suspected "KS virus" are underway.[19] The most popular AIDS drug, AZT, has been discredited, and physicians are reduced to offering their HIV Positive patients the experimental drug (or "cocktail") of the moment on a "try it, you might like it" basis. Many of these drugs are highly toxic, especially when combined, and their "side-effects" read like a list of AIDS symptoms. In short, things are a mess. Meanwhile, the AIDS conveyor belt rolls on, providing employment for an ever-increasing army of support personnel. And every week, the roll of sick and dying young men grows longer.[20]

---

[19]John Lauritsen, "NIDA Meeting Calls For Research Into The Poppers-Kaposi's Sarcoma Connection". See Appendix B.

[20]As of 1996, the incidence of AIDS among drug addicts and the very poor is rising; among gay men it is apparently on the downswing. In the future, will the majority of gay men with AIDS be young men who have repeatedly practised "unsafe sex" and, after seroconversion, taken toxic medications? A recent study conducted at St. Mary's Hospital, London, compared two groups of patients recently diagnosed with AIDS. One group had tested HIV Positive up to eight years previously, and had been attending the clinic and taking prescribed medications. The other group had not previously been tested and

Gay men have long served as repositories for a complex of group fears and fantasies about sex, sickness and death. Psychohistorian Lloyd deMause has drawn attention to society's periodic killing off of "its own id-representatives, its youth, who represent itself in the life-phase when it was most sexual and most aggressive."[21] In the past, this filicidal syndrome has usually been acted out through war. The frequent employment of war metaphors in AIDS literature of all kinds suggests that in the Eighties and Nineties, AIDS is taking the place of war, or has become a new kind of war.[22] Under the veneer of a compassionate liberalism, psychobiochemical assault is being inflicted on gay men: not as a conscious intention, but as the result of policies predicated on certain unconsciously held ideas.

It is time to rethink this crisis, to begin to understand how we might extricate ourselves from the nightmare that has overtaken us, and enveloped us now for almost two decades. We will not understand the phenomenon of the seroconvert until we begin to investigate the destructive hold of unconscious belief systems in which we all participate. Until then, all the AIDS Education and Safe Sex Information in the world will not prevent new cohorts of young men from summoning up their courage and heading from the Test Site to the tattoo parlor to take up their cross.

---

had taken no AIDS medications. The unmedicated group was healthier.

[21]Lloyd deMause, "Historical Group-Fantasies" in *Foundations of Psychohistory,* New York, Creative Roots, 1982, p. 192.

[22]For a further discussion of this process, see Young, *op. cit.*

Appendix A

AIDS Criticism: Books, Articles, and Other Resources

The following list of AIDS-criticism resources is intended to be brief and selective:

Organizations and Publications:

Continuum was founded in 1992 as a pro-life organization for those who are or want to be long-term survivors of an "HIV-positive" or an "AIDS" diagnosis. The group publishes an outstanding bimonthly magazine, which is on the cutting edge of AIDS criticism — questioning not only the HIV-AIDS hypothesis and the orthodox (and lethal) AIDS medications, but the very existence of HIV as an infectious, exogenous virus. Continuum can be reached at: 172 Foundling Court, Brunswick Centre, London WC1N 1QE, England. Tel.: [+44] 171 713-7071.

The Group for the Scientific Reappraisal of the HIV-AIDS Hypothesis, founded by Charles A. Thomas, Jr., includes several hundred scientists and other professionals: 7514 Girard Ave., #1-331, La Jolla, CA 92037. Telephone: (619) 272-1621.

HEAL (Health Education AIDS Liaison) has provided alternative AIDS information for over a decade, and now has branches in a number of different cities and countries. For information contact the head branch in New York City: P.O. Box 1103, Old Chelsea Station, New York, NY 10113. Telephone: 212 873-0780.

Positively Healthy have been helping those with "AIDS" or "HIV-positive" diagnoses to return to health and stay healthy since the late 80s: Positively Healthy, P.O. Box 71, Richmond, Surrey TW9 3DJ, ENGLAND. Telephone: [+44] 181 878-6443.

Internet Web Sites:

Rethinking AIDS: http://www.xs4all.nl/~raido/
Sumeria: http://www.livelinks.com/sumeria/
HEAL: http://www.aidsnyc.org/heal/
The AIDS Information BBS:
By gopher: gopher://itsa.ucsf.edu:70/00/.i/.q/.d/
By ftp: ftp ftp://itsa/ucsf/edu:70/00/.i/.q/.d/
By web: http://itsa.ucsf.edu/~beng/aidsbbs.html

Books and Articles:

Peter H. Duesberg (editor).
AIDS: Virus or Drug Induced?
Articles by E. Papadopulos-Eleopulos et al., P. Duesberg, V. Koliadin, M. Craddock, M. Zaretsky, D. Chiu, R. Root-Bernstein, H. Haverkos, D. Drotman, B. Ellison, A. Downey, G. Stewart, K. Mullis, S. Harris, S. Lang, N. Hodgkinson, P. Johnson, T. Bethell, J. Lauritsen, and C. Farber.
Kluwer Academics Press, Dordrecht, The Netherlands 1996.

Peter H. Duesberg.
Infectious AIDS: Have We Been Misled?.
A collection of thirteen articles originally published in scientific journals.
North Atlantic Books (1996).

Peter H. Duesberg.
Inventing The AIDS Virus.
Regnery Publishing, Inc. (1996).

HEAL (Health Education AIDS Liaison).
Comprehensive Information Packet.
(See above.)

Neville Hodgkinson.
AIDS: The Failure of Contemporary Science.
Fourth Estate (1996).

John Lauritsen.
The AIDS War: Propaganda, Profiteering and Genocide from the Medical-Industrial Complex.
Asklepios (1993).

Eleni Papadopulos-Eleopulos, Valendar F. Turner. and John M. Papadimitriou.
"Is a Western Blot Proof of HIV Infection?".
Bio/Technology, June 1993, pp. 691-707.

Charles A. Thomas Jr., Kary B. Mullis, and Phillip E. Johnson.
"What Causes AIDS: It's an Open Question".
Reason, June 1994. (The December 1994 issue of REASON has 10 pages devoted to correspondence and authors' replies concerning the June article.)

Ian Young.
The AIDS Dissidents: An Annotated Bibliography.
The Scarecrow Press (1993)

Appendix B

Toxicities of Poppers (Nitrite Inhalants) A Brief Bibliography

Books:

Harry W. Haverkos and John A. Dougherty (editors).
Health Hazards of Nitrite Inhalants.
NIDA Research Monograph 83, 1988.
National Institute on Drug Abuse.

John Lauritsen and Hank Wilson.
Death Rush: Poppers & AIDS.
New York 1986.
(out-of-print)

Articles:

E.M. Dax, W.H. Adler, *et al.*
"Amyl Nitrite Alters Human In Vitro Immune Function".
Immunopharmacology and Immunotoxicology.
13(4), 577-587 (1991).

Adi A. Gerblich, Ann E. Campbell, *et al.*
"Changes in T-cell Lymphocyte Subpopulations After Antigenic Bronchial Provocation in Asthmatics".
New England Journal of Medicine, May 1984.

David A. Guss, Sven A. Normann, *et al.*
"Clinically Significant Methemoglobinemia from Inhalation of Isobutyl Nitrite".
American Journal of Emergency Medicine, January 1985.

Thomas H. Haley.
"Review of the Physiological Effects of Amyl, Butyl, and Isobutyl Nitrites".
Clinical Toxicology, pp. 317-329, 1980.

Evan M. Hersh, James M. Reuben, *et al.*
"Effect of the Recreational Agent Isobutyl Nitrite on Human Blood Leukocytes and on in Vitro Interferon Production".
Cancer Research, March 1983.

McDonald K. Horne, III, Michael R. Waterman, *et al.*
"Methemoglobinemia from Sniffing Butyl Nitrite".
Annals of Internal Medicine, September 1979.

Richard F. Jacobs, Daniel J. Marmer, *et al.*
"Cellular Immunotoxicity of Amyl Nitrite".
Journal of Toxicology- Clinical Toxicology, pp. 421-449 (1983).

Karl A. Jørgensen and Sven-Olov Lawesson.
"Amyl Nitrite and Kaposi's Sarcoma in Homosexual Men".
New England Journal of Medicine, 30 September 1982.

John Lauritsen.
"NIDA Meeting Calls For Research Into The Poppers-Kaposi's Sarcoma Connection".
New York Native, issue 582, 13 June 1994.

On the Rethinking AIDS and Sumeria web sites. See Appendix A.

Eva Lotzovà, Cherylyn A. Savary, *et al.*
"Depression of Murine Natural Killer Cell Cytotoxicity by Isobutyl Nitrite".
Cancer Immunology Immunotherapy, pp. 130-134, vol. 17, 1984.

D.J. Marmer, R.F. Jacobs, *et al.*
"In Vitro Immunotoxicity of Amyl Nitrite".
Clinical Research, vol. 30, no. 5, 1982.

M.J. Morgan, A.S. Kimes and E.D. London.
"Possible Roles for Nitric Oxide in AIDS and Associated Pathology".
Medical Hypotheses (1992) 38, 189-193.

J.R. Neefe, A. Ganjii, *et al.*
"Daily Amyl Nitrite Inhalation Decreases Mouse Splenocyte Response to Concanavalin A".
Federation Proceedings 42 (abstract 3850), 5 March 1983.

Guy R. Newell, Stephen C. Adams, *et al.*
"Toxicity, Immunosuppressive Effects and Carcinogenic Potential of volatile Nitrites: Possible relationship to Kaposi's Sarcoma".
Pharmacotherapy, September 1984.

Jesse S. Ortiz and Vilma L. Rivera.
"The Effect of Amyl Nitrite on T-Cell Function in Mice".
(Presentation to the American Public Health Association convention, November 1985).
Reprinted in Haverkos, *op. cit.*

J. Osterloh and D. Goldfield.
"Butyl Nitrite Transformation in Vitro, Chemical Nitrosation Reactions, and Mutagenesis".
Journal of Analytical Toxicology, July / August 1984.

I. Quinto.
"The Mutagenicity of Alkylnitrites in the Salmonella test".
(Translation from the Italian).
Bolletino Società Italiana Biologia Sperimentale, 1980, 56:816-820.

K.R. Romeril and A.J. Concannon.
"Heinz Body Haemolytic Anaemia after Sniffing Volatile Nitrites".
The Medical Journal of Australia, March 1981.

Lee S.F. Soderberg and John B. Barnett.
"Exposure to Inhaled Isobutyl Nitrite Reduces T Cell Blastogenesis and Antibody Responsiveness".
Fundamental and Applied Toxicology 17, 821-824 (1991).

Lee S.F. Soderberg, James Flick and John B. Barnett.
"Acute inhalation exposure to isobutyl nitrite causes nonspecific blood cell destruction".
Experimental Hematology 24:592-596 (1996).

Lee S.F. Soderberg, James Flick and John B. Barnett.
"Leukopenia and altered hematopoietic activity in mice exposed to the abused inhalant, isobutyl nitrite".
Experimental Hematology 24:848-853 (1996).

Colophon

The text font for this book is Dante, designed by Giovanni Mardersteig — an outstanding scholar of printing, as well as one of the leading typographers of the 20th century. Cut in 1954, Dante was Dr. Mardersteig's last and finest type. It is an original design, strongly influenced by fifteenth century Italian typefaces.

In his book, *Anatomy of a Typeface*, Alexander Lawson devotes an entire chapter to Mardersteig. He describes Dante in the following terms:

> Although produced for a private press, Dante is by no means over-refined, a condemnation that may be applied to so many types of similar conception. As a book type it has few idiosyncrasies to interfere with its readability. Its crisp and sparkling contrast of stroke is eminently suited both to the antique finish of most book papers and to the dull-coated stocks, used for illustrations.... The italic is a chancery, matching beautifully the spirit of the roman.

This version of Dante was supplied in Postscript form by Monotype Corporation.

The font on the covers and spine is Plantin, designed for Monotype by F.H. Pierpoint, whose model was a typeface of the eminent sixteenth century Antwerp printer, Christophe Plantin.

The book was produced on a Gateway2000 486 PC, using WordPerfect 5.1 for DOS and Prime Type. It was printed on an HP-Laserjet IIIP.